MW00655852

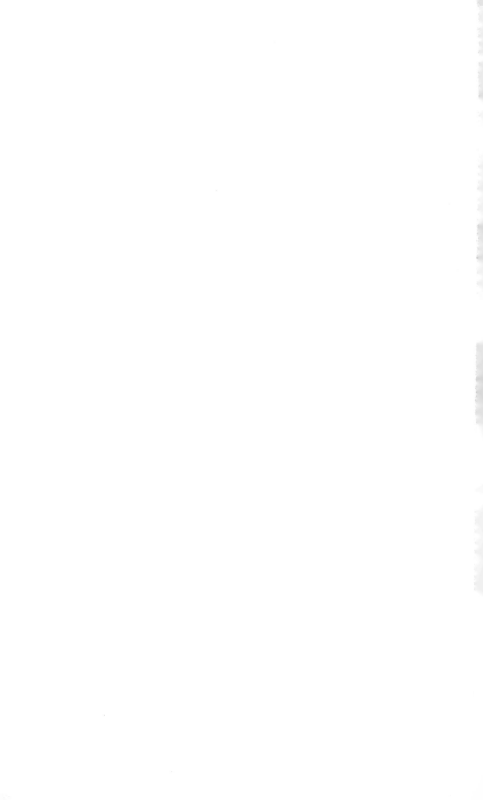

What others have to say about this book:

"That Guy Nurse" has written a lucid, insightful book that looks at health in a meaningful, practical way. It makes me reevaluate my own life and health. It brings in philosophy and humor, yet hits home.

Louann Biccick, Professor of Nursing
Marian College, Fond du Lac, Wisconsin

The efforts of ThatGuyNurse, which have reached hundreds of thousands across the country, are changing the course of history and are changing the course of health care.

Notes from ThatGuyNurse: Choose Today Live Tomorrow *should be a must read for clinicians, policymakers, advocates, and consumers alike. It is more than a provocative commentary on the "highs" and "lows" of the U.S. health care delivery system. It is an up-close and personal account of medical care as it is today. And it is a charge and challenge to clinicians, administrators, and policymakers to build a system that truly supports health promotion, disease prevention, and health care.*

The insights articulated relative to health promotion, disease prevention, evidence-based practice, and informed decisionmaking extend even further the adage, "Give a man a fish and he eats for a day. Teach him to fish and he eats for a lifetime." The vision is clear. If we learn and adopt the lessons prescribed across the life cycle, we could potentially almost eradicate sickness.

Sandra Millon Underwood RN, PhD, FAAN
Professor, University of Wisconsin Milwaukee
College of Nursing

Notes from
ThatGuyNurse:
Choose Today, Live Tomorrow

For more information and copies of
this book, please contact:
www.thatguynurse.com

Published by:
9th Street Publishing
154 N. Broadway, Green Bay, WI 54303

Cover Design and Layout by: Prophit Marketing
www.prophitmarketing.com

Manufactured in the United States of America

Notes from ThatGuyNurse:
Choose Today, Live Tomorrow

by
John D. Shier RN, PhD
thatguynurse.com

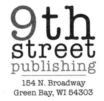
9th
street
publishing
154 N. Broadway
Green Bay, WI 54303

Notes from ThatGuyNurse
Choose Today, Live Tomorrow

by: John Shier, RN, PhD

Contents

About ThatGuyNurse

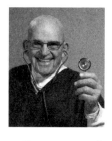 I'm currently a registered nurse living in Green Bay, Wisconsin, and in this book I'll be sharing some of the many things I have learned as a nurse. First, some background.

I grew up in Madison, Wisconsin. My mother was a registered nurse. Only when I became a registered nurse fairly late in life did I discover what it meant to be a nurse and how much the education I received in my nursing studies differed from the training she received in the 1920s. For mom, the primary role of the nurse was to provide comfort. She was of a generation of nurses who were unfairly but not inappropriately described as "pillow plumpers." She was a nurse before hospitals were the primary venue for patient care. Her nursing was largely done in patient homes and largely involved activities that are today assigned to nursing assistants: bathing patients, feeding patients, and sitting at the bedside to provide comfort.

Mom died before I entered nursing school, but I would have loved to have been able for the two of us to share our nursing experiences and to discover how, although I was trained in a world of technical complexity and sophistication she could not imagine, as nurses we still shared a fundamental commitment to patient care.

I graduated from St. Olaf, a small Lutheran college in Minnesota, a very long time ago. Following college I served in the Navy for four years as an anti-submarine air intelligence officer and then returned to graduate school at the University of Wisconsin–Madison. I received my master's and doctoral degrees in philosophy and began my adult life as a professor of philosophy there.

In 1965, my wonderful wife, Rosalie, and I moved to Green Bay, where I was part of the team that started the University of Wisconsin–Green Bay. I loved teaching very much and did it for many years. When an opportunity came to go out into the real world, though, I took it. For four years, I was the Executive Director of the Northeastern Wisconsin Area Agency on Aging, a federally funded organization that advocated for older Americans. Following that I spent 14 years as the Executive Director of the Brown County (Green Bay) United Way. Being the boss wasn't too shabby.

But then, in 1982, my best friend, Ron, who lived in Rockford, Illinois, called, saying, "John, something's wrong. I'm scared. Can you come?" I went to Rockford to find that, at age 47, my best friend had liver cancer. I stayed with him. Gratefully, it was a kind of cancer that did not cause a

About thatguynurse

lot of pain, but in six weeks he was dead. I had never been through that kind of experience before, and when I returned to Green Bay, I found myself drawn to the local hospice program.

In 1982, I became a hospice volunteer. For the next 10 years, I found myself spending more and more time doing hospice work. Hospice is a program for people who are dying. They have cancer or heart disease or diabetes or some other illness that is both progressive and that has gone beyond the point where cure is possible. The remainder of life is measured in a few months or weeks. Our job in hospice was to help the patient, and often the family, deal with the pain and even the terror that can accompany dying. I was trained to do patient care, most often going into a home to spend the night so that the primary caregiver could get some badly needed rest.

For 10 years, I became more and more deeply involved in being a hospice volunteer, and in 1992, I asked Rosalie for permission to resign from my job so that I could return to college to study nursing. In retrospect, she was clearly delighted to get me out of the house. "What a wonderful idea," she said. "Please do it!"

I packed up, left Green Bay, and moved into Sandburg dorms at the University of Wisconsin–Milwaukee. Dorm life had changed from that of a little Lutheran College in Minnesota in the 1950s. All for the better, I might add. I was enrolled in an accelerated nursing program designed for students who had already received a bachelor's degree. The program required taking at least 19 credits each semester and 13 credits during two summers. It was intense and required full time for study. At UWM, as it is known, you are expected to party every weekend. And so, every four weeks or so I would take my laundry home to Rosalie. It was a great life!

In nursing school, we formed study groups; invaluable tools for dealing with the complex studies of anatomy, physiology, pharmacology, nursing diagnoses, and dozens of other subjects. We practiced nursing skills on one another. One of the most interesting skills involved needles and syringes for drawing blood, for starting intravenous injections (IVs), and/or giving injections subcutaneously (just under the skin) or intramuscularly (deep into the flesh). To learn these skills, the nursing program provided us with practice artificial arms, legs, and torsos. These practice body parts had been used by hundreds of prior nursing students. Little skill was needed to decide where to put the needle, as the dummies had been perforated thousands of times before we got them and had needle tracks that would make a junkie proud.

Thus, my dorm room became the laboratory we couldn't

About thatguynurse

have at school. Syringes and alcohol swabs would disappear from school and reemerge in my room, where we would practice on each other. Woe to the person who had "great veins": veins that stood out like garden hoses. They were termed "easy sticks" and spent most of the semester with black-and-blue arms and long sleeves to keep the secret from the professors.

As a guy nursing student and quite a bit older than the rest of my colleagues, I learned a lesson that I think most women had learned for a very long time in the men's world: I had to do twice as much and do it twice as well as the woman nurses just to be considered competent. Any error would bring forth comments like, "Well, that's a man for you," or "That must have been a senior moment." A professor once made a joke: "Why did God create Adam before Eve? Because He wanted to practice to be sure He got it right."

The study of nursing did not come easy for a philosopher though. Courses in chemistry, physics, organic chemistry, microbiology, anatomy, physiology, and genetics—just to name a few—were difficult. It was a struggle, but I graduated from the College of Nursing in 1995. I had finished college again! That was a special time for me: I got to start what has turned out to be a wonderful third career and I turned 60 all in the same month.

After my return to Green Bay, I took a position as a staff nurse at the hospice where I had volunteered for so many years; I also took a second position on the cardiac floor of a local hospital. For much of the last 16 years, I've been a hospice nurse and a cardiac nurse.

It wasn't long after I started nursing that I became aware that something has gone terribly and horribly wrong with the American medical system. I can't remember if I was in intensive care with a fresh open-heart or lung resection or out on the cardiac floor or in a hospice home, but it was clear to me that something had gone wrong. In the hospital patients were trying to deal with degrees of pain and fear and massive expense that I could not even imagine. In the hospice homes they were dying, and their dying often took a long, hard, suffering time to accomplish. Something said to me that it's not supposed to be this way. There shouldn't be this much fear and pain and expense in getting through life.

So I did what philosophers do. We do try to make sense of things that do not seem to make very much sense. And so for some years, I've tried to make sense out of the American medical system. In this book, I will share my thoughts with you.

About thatguynurse

Why "thatguynurse" ?

In 2000, I did a presentation I called "To Live Long and To Die Healthy" at a Green Bay company whose president was a good friend and very interested in helping to keep his employees healthy. A friend of his who owned a trucking company heard about the program and asked if I would do some audiotapes to send out to his 15,000 drivers. I arranged to spend a week riding a semi truck around the country to find out what life was like on the road. Then I began doing monthly segments about being healthy on the road that went to all the drivers. Just a few months later I got a call from the company. They rarely heard from their drivers, but now they were getting calls asking for some more information from "that guy nurse." Now, more than 1700 presentations later to more than 300 corporations, I am proud to be "thatguynurse."

Often when people find out that I am a philosopher, they shrug and say, "I took a course in philosophy when I was in college. I didn't understand a thing." The question of what it is that philosophers do is a mystery to a great many people. So, then, what is it that philosophers do? Generally they try to look at the world from new and different perspectives. Remember when we as children would look up at the clouds and imagine that they looked like something. "Oh, look, there's a horse!" "No! It's a fish!" The world is sort of like that. Whatever it really is, we can see it in many different ways. Thus, when I look at the world of medicine from the standpoint of being a nurse, I don't see a "health care" system. What I see is a "medical" system. I see a system whose goal is to cure disease and to repair trauma. I do not see a health care system whose goal is to help patients maintain good health throughout their lives.

How we see things does make a difference. Consider the transformation of life and society that occurred when Galileo suggested that we look at the world as being Sun-centered rather than seeing the Earth as the center of the universe." To us, it is impossible to imagine the sun as being the center of the universe or to imagine, as the ancients did, that the world is flat and resting on the back of an elephant that, in turn, stands on a turtle. Now imagine how the world might look to people a thousand years from now and how they might, looking back, think how primitive our view of the world was.

Seeing the world of medicine as being focused on cure and repair rather than on health can help each of us to understand that we have both the opportunity and the responsibility for our own health. And since health is the most important thing we have, we have to focus on how we can use the medical system in such ways that we make it, for each of us, a genuine health care system. That is what this book is all about.

Acknowledgements

I could not be alive and doing what I do if it not for a wonderful lady, Rosalie. She is my wife. She has been with me for 50 years. She has supported me through success and failure for all of that time. I could not ask for anybody better, more loyal or more loving. Thank you.

Rosalie and I have a daughter, Elizabeth. She is an artist a creative person. She seeks and loves adventure. She inspires me every moment of every day. Thank you.

I entered the University of Wisconsin–Milwaukee College of Nursing in 1992, where my first professor was Dr. Sandra Millon-Underwood. From the moment of our first class together, she inspired me to be a nurse. To be a nurse, she said, was to be a teacher. I have tried to fulfill her challenge. Thank you.

Eight years ago I met a doctor, Daniel Garrison Koster, MD. He is brilliant, everything that I believe a doctor should be. He has inspired me to write this book. Thank you.

Way back in 1982, the people at Unity Hospice gave me the opportunity to be a volunteer. That experience turned my life around. Their support, coaching, and encouragement made it possible for me to become a nurse. Thank you.

I have an assistant, Kathy McKenzie. She keeps me honest.

She represents me and is the foundation of all that I have experienced as "thatguynurse." Almost everybody assumes (and they are correct) that she is my boss. Thank you.

When I felt I was ready to have my thoughts put into print, it was recommended that I contact Carolyn Kott Washburne to be my editor. I did. What you are about to read is in so many way the result of her coaching, directing, leading, and giving my written words my "voice." Thank you.

Finally, for over more than 26 years, it has been my honor to be with hundreds of patients in hospice and in the hospital. Each and every one of them has given me something that I could never repay, a feeling of joy at being alive and a feeling of gratitude that I could make a gift to another human being.

John D. Shier RN, PhD
thatguynurse

Welcome to this Book!

It sounds incredible, and you may believe it belies immodesty on the part of the author to say it, but this is probably the most important book you'll ever read. Why? Because if you are between 18 and 60 years of age as you are reading this, YOU will probably live to the age of 90 to 100 years. That's right—I said 100 years.

The challenge, I've learned, is to live in good health throughout that time. I wrote this book because in my years of nursing experience, including 10-plus years as a hospice nurse, it has become alarmingly apparent that each of us, individually, will make key decisions in our own lifetimes that determine whether the last 30 years of our lifetimes are absolutely miserable or fantastically active, exciting, and productive.

How do you ensure that your lifetime, the full span of your lifetime, is time spent healthy, active, and engaged in the activities of the world? Reading this book and applying the basic principles within these covers is an excellent start. This means learning about and understanding the conditions of health. It also means assuming a whole new dimension of personal responsibility for your health—and that's where this book comes in.

The good news is that within the lifetimes of many of

us, advances in medical science have virtually eliminated many of the historical causes of death. Numerous diseases, once lethal, either no longer exist or are easily treatable—measles, mumps, diphtheria, tuberculosis, polio, and scarlet fever, to name a few. Trauma care and surgical interventions have advanced to the point where the injuries and systemic failures that were once invariably fatal can now be remedied.

The troubling news, however, is that the current American medical system of hospitals, clinics, physicians, nurses, and technicians, insurance companies, pharmaceutical companies, and equipment manufacturers is not a real "health care" system. It is, rather, a "sickness care" system. Few of the billions of dollars invested in medical care today go to the creation and maintenance of health. The primary focus of medical care is to keep patients alive—whether they want to be or not.

In other words, those who are chronically ill with diabetes, lung cancer, heart disease, arthritis, or illnesses related to obesity or any of a number of other conditions will still live nearly to the full extent of that 90-to-100-year projected life span, but their years will be filled with medications, procedures, tests, hospital stays, pain, and the gradual elimination of all of the activities they enjoyed throughout life.

That Guy Nurse

What You'll Find in this Book

To provide a little background, in Part I of this book, "Five Rules for Long-Term Health," I look at the impact of the medical system and how it has extended life expectancy in the United States from age 54 in the 1930s to nearly 80 today. I also emphasize the critical fact that the American medical system provides medical practitioners few financial incentives for health—it is a system designed to cure sickness and to repair trauma and to keep patients alive.

There is a lot of criticism of the American health care system, particularly of the degree to which the quest for profit creates conflicts of interest throughout the system, conflicts in which the patient often comes off the worse for wear. There is also criticism of patients who because of ignorance or fear misuse the system and thereby both place themselves at risk and drive up the already unsupportable costs of American health care.

As a result—and this is the part that I can't emphasize enough to you, my readers—is that it is up to each one of us to do what is necessary to build and maintain good health. Through personal lifestyle decisions you can—and must—take primary responsibility for the maintenance of your health through the full human life span of 90 to 100 years. In the final chapter of Part I lay down some guidelines for how to do this.

Part II, "The Professional Patient: How to Make the

Welcome to This Book!

System Work for You," emphasizes, first, that you are the president and CEO of your own life. I show you how to take charge! In the 21st century, patients and physicians must become partners, working together and sharing knowledge. This section also describes how to choose a physician to be your coach and mentor.

Part III, "Issues and Decisions at the End of Life," might be difficult for some of you to read, but it's essential. Death and dying aren't like they used to be, and if you don't ask yourself the tough questions—and share the answers with your loved ones and health care professionals—you'll lose control over the process. I know from my hospice work that this isn't pretty.

Finally, I can't resist getting on my soapbox for a bit. In Part IV, "A Vision for the Future of Medical Practice in the U.S.," I spell how the American medical system must change. It will become a true "wellness system" only when patients assume responsibility for their own health and learn to use the skills of physicians, nurses, and others in the medical system as vehicles for health rather than as mechanics who fix the things that go wrong. The focus of the new system will be on prevention of disease and trauma and on the maintenance of health.

What This Book Is and What It Is Not

This is not a how-to book. This is not the place to go if you want specifics on how to exercise or how to eat. There is no expansive bibliography of reference books to provide all of that information. During my years as a university professor, I came to draw a distinction between those of my colleagues whom I thought of as "tellers" and those whom I thought of as "teachers." Tellers were people who through long years of study and long years of learning had acquired lots of information about English literature or Physics or Medieval poetry. They regarded their task as professors to be that of telling the students all the things that they had learned and then expecting the students to put that information down on exams. Teachers, on the other hand, gave the students the information they needed to be able to go out into the world and find the things they needed to know. The teachers enabled students to continue in and to direct their own courses of learning. Perhaps this is to make the distinction in the old saying, "Give a man a fish and he eats for a day. Teach him how to fish and he eats for a lifetime."

I hope that this can be a teaching book. If some of the ideas expressed here strike you as interesting or important I hope you will feel motivated to go on the Internet or to the library or bookstore and learn about exercise and nutrition, stress management, and the medical system and how to confront the challenges that arise as you or a loved one comes to the end of life.

Welcome to This Book!

The American Medical System: Something Has Gone Terribly Wrong

How to use this book:

[In Chapter IV, I'll share with you the Five Key Elements of Long-Term Health. If you're glancing through this book for a "quick and dirty" understanding of my message, you're welcome to skip to Chapter 5. But I invite you to read the four preceding chapters to know the philosophic underpinnings of my message.]

Few topics are more widely discussed or of greater concern in the United States than the cost and quality of medical care. These topics are central in the conversations of corporate executives and third-shift workers. They are central in political discourse and in dinner conversations.

2009 was the year of "Health Care Reform." A legislative proposal to alter radically the structure and operation of the American health care system dominated the nation's interest for a year and beyond. It spawned both hopes and fears across the country. It created a spate of rumors and outright falsehoods as both its opponents and supporters fought by any means possible to win the day for their point of view. Finally it led to politically motivated compromises that virtually gutted its most important provisions. And the minute that Congress passed a bill calling for sweeping changes in how medical care is organized and delivered, there began a movement to have the entire bill repealed.

This is nothing new in America and it should not be surprising. For the better part of a century, every president has attempted to reform American's medical system. And all of their efforts have been frustrated.

Coalitions, primarily consisting of insurance companies, pharmaceutical companies, companies that manufacture medical equipment, physicians' associations and hospital corporations, have successfully convinced the American public that any alternative to the current American medical system would be disastrous in terms of both cost and care. As of this writing, it is not clear that the proposed reforms of 2010 will ultimately be enacted. Yet there is almost unanimous agreement across the country that the American medical system is broken and in need of major repair even though there is little agreement on how the fix should be accomplished.

There is good reason for this consensus on the dysfunction of the medical system. The cost of medical care in the United States is the leading cause of personal and family bankruptcy.[1] Some 40 million Americans have no medical insurance. Many of them have chosen not to pay for medical insurance, but a great number are those who either cannot afford it or are disqualified because of a prior medical condition. Yet even as millions of Americans without medical insurance live in fear of illness, and while millions more worry that they'll lose their insurance, the majority of Americans continue to believe that the United States has the finest health care system in the world. Part of this belief relates to the idea that America must be the very best in everything. Part of it, though, relates to some widely held yet erroneous beliefs about the health care system and how it operates. We will explore these beliefs and attendant attitudes in later chapters.

The topic of health care reform dominates much of the political debate among candidates for state and national office. Through Medicare and Medicaid, our government is hugely affected by the ruinously escalating costs of medicine. Our tax dollars directly pay for medical care in two main ways. First, Medicare must cover medical costs for a rapidly growing population of older Americans with expensive, chronic conditions. Second, government programs now pay

---

[1]   http://www.nchc.org/facts/cost.shtml

The American Medical System:
Something Has Gone Terribly Wrong

A Medical "Save"

Before I went to nursing school, I had to take a lot of science courses that I had managed to avoid during college. It took two full semesters and summer school to finish 42 credits of sciences. Physics, introduction to chemistry, bio-organic chemistry, microbiology, anatomy, physiology, and genetics were required courses to gain entrance to the College of Nursing. Facing all of that and hoping to earn some income while I pursued my nursing studies, I took a six-week course that certified me as a Nursing Assistant.

My first assignment was for a child. Billy (not his real name) was seven years old. He lived with foster parents. His mother apparently used a lot of cocaine while she was pregnant. Billy continues to pay a price for her habit. He had, in essence, no brain in his skull. He had the lower brain, sometimes called the reptilian brain, whose function is to control heartbeat and respiration. Billy was blind and deaf. He could not speak. He was incapable of voluntarily moving his arms or his legs. He could not swallow and so had a feeding tube inserted through the wall of his abdomen and into his stomach. Billy's nervous system was incapable of controlling his temperature, and so whenever he became too warm, clothes would be removed. When he became chilled, clothing was added.

During my brief time working with Billy, I would arrive at his home at 6:30 a.m. His foster mother would have given him his morning tube feeding and dressed him. Billy would be lying on the living room carpet, very still and quiet. About seven o'clock a specially equipped van would arrive, and Billy and I would board the van, Billy in a wheelchair. My job was to escort him to a special school for severely handicapped children. Being blind and deaf and incapable of speech or movement, Billy was not able to participate in any of the educational offerings of the school.

28

> Rather, he was in essence warehoused for the day.
>
> At 3:30 p.m., I would arrive at his home and meet the bus to drive to school. Once again he would be loaded onto the bus in his wheelchair and returned to his home. Once home, I would feed him via the feeding tube and then carry him into the bathroom, where I would hold him suspended over the commode until he urinated and defecated. I would then lay him down on the living room carpet, where he would lie quiet and motionless.
>
> Billy had been "saved" by a very high-tech, critical care unit of the hospital where he was born. For the first year of his life, highly skilled doctors and nurses attended him. Then he was turned over to his foster parents, who were provided with a specially equipped van for transportation as well as financial support for his clothing, feeding tube supplies, and other treatments. In addition to the care of his foster parents, he required the support, every morning and evening, seven days a week, of nurses and nursing assistants.
>
> It has been years since I saw Billy. He may well still be alive at 21, still in the care of foster parents and support staff.

for younger Americans who survived, often with extensive, expensive treatments, medical conditions that were fatal to infants or children a couple of generations ago. Consider infants born with Down syndrome, cerebral palsy, or cystic fibrosis. In the middle of the 20th century, these children had life expectancies measured in weeks to several years. Now, with the advent of antibiotics and specialized nursing, respiratory care, and other care, these people often live into their 50s.

The American Medical System:
Something Has Gone Terribly Wrong

Almost everyone has experienced, either personally or through family or friends, the miracles of American health care. And the same is true for the horrors of American health care. Generally, though, discussion centers on the horrors: prescription errors, long struggles with insurance companies, misdiagnoses, the constant changing of physicians as employers opt for a cheaper form of coverage, patients missing necessary treatments due to lack of insurance. On and on and on the stories go, and many, mostly older, Americans yearn for that time not so long ago when doctors and patients knew each other well, when the doctor was seen as a friend as well as a healer, and when medical bills could be paid in loaves of bread or sides of beef. But, of course, that time exists largely in imagination. As one man said, "The main thing about the good old days is that they weren't."[2] That golden time in the past is probably as exaggerated as many of today's tales of medical horror. But somewhere between those dreamy old golden days and our modern medical nightmares, you will find the true state of affairs. And the truth is that the American medical system is broken—terribly broken and with no apparent repair in sight.

---

[2] In every age "the good old days" were a myth. No one ever thought they were good at the time. For every age has consisted of crises that seemed intolerable to the people who lived through them. — Brooks Atkinson (1894 - 1984), *Once Around the Sun* (1951)

That Guy Nurse

The Good Ol' Days—and Today

There was a time when the term "family doctor" meant someone who knew every member of the family, often from the cradle to the grave. There was a time when one could approach the doctor or even hospitalization without the fear of massive bills. That was a time when grown children tended to stay in the same community rather than spreading themselves across the continent. By remaining close, families were capable of providing support when a member became sick or injured. That was a time when death came quickly after a brief illness or accident, and the doctor was there to comfort the dying patient and the grieving family. That time was probably the golden age of the patient-doctor relationship, when the doctor was known and trusted for years by the community he served.

Yet, consider this—one of the key points in this book. That golden age of the doctor-patient relationship was a time when the physician was practically powerless in dealing with most health threats. At a time when the doctor was your closest ally in the fight for survival, he had very few weapons against the wide variety of illnesses, infections, and injuries that ended lives and brought suffering. Most of what we now consider minor inconveniences were then potential killers. But doctors did their best with what weapons they had. Sometimes all they could do was be there. There was much

The American Medical System:
Something Has Gone Terribly Wrong

that was wonderful and worth remembering about that time, but there was also much we are glad to leave behind.

Death tended to come early a century ago. Life expectancy was still only 54 around 1950. Many people did live well into their 80s and 90s in those days, but they were the lucky ones. Millions died in infancy and childhood from myriad diseases. They died from measles, mumps, diphtheria, tuberculosis, polio, scarlet fever, and a host of other diseases that either

The Corn Chopper Miracle

Some years ago I admitted a 72-year-old farmer to hospice. He died of lung cancer because he was a smoker and that's what smokers tend to die from. As I did the physical assessment required for his admission, I discovered that completely encircling the top of his right arm was a scar, the most horrendous a scar I have ever seen. I asked him what happened. He responded, "Oh, about seven or eight years ago my son I were a working out there in the south field. I got my arm caught in the corn chopper." It severed his arm. Sliced it off! At any other time or place in history this man would have been dead where he dropped. Not now, though. His son reached into the tractor and pulled out a cell phone. He punched 911. A medical helicopter came to the farm, picked up the farmer and his arm, and took them back to the hospital, where the arm was reattached. It never did work very well. But the man did not die of shock. He did not die of infection. He did not die of blood loss. He died of lung cancer because he was a smoker.

That Guy Nurse

no longer exist or, at worst, make one sick for a few days. People died of infections spreading from simple cuts on a leg, foot, or hand. They died of injuries as simple as a broken leg from which a blood clot moved into the lungs because medical science had not yet come up with blood thinners. Everyone knew about quarantines for diseases like scarlet fever, measles, and mumps, and every city or county had a hospital solely for patients with tuberculosis.

It Is Very Hard to Die! Hold on to this Thought!

Further, beginning in the 1950s, we began to create surgical technologies of unbelievable sophistication. I am a cardiac nurse. At my hospital, we do an average of 15 open-heart surgeries each week. "Open-heart surgery," also known as "coronary artery bypass graft surgery," or "CABBAGE," is one of the most-performed surgeries in the United States. But nobody ever woke up in the morning and said, "Geeze, it's cold, it's rainy, and I'm bored. I think I'll have open-heart surgery." No.

People have open-heart surgery when their heart disease is so advanced that they are going to die. They are probably already on cardiac medications. They probably have already had an angioplasty. They may have stents holding one or more coronary arteries open. But their heart disease has advanced, and unless they come in and surgeons open their chest and sew new arteries on their heart, they are dead. As a result, millions of Americans are walking the streets with that railroad track scar down their chests. Forty years ago they were all dead.[3]

Modern American medicine, with all of its problems, nevertheless can cure illnesses and injuries that would have brought death 50 years ago. But these miracles come at a price. We all want the benefits of modern medicine, but most of us struggle with the costs, both financial and personal. Does our American medical system provide its miracles at a fair price? Or, perhaps a better question is, what can Americans do to gain these—and even greater miracles—for less?

Historically, to be a patient was to be under the care of a physician. The patient's role was to present his or her symptoms and to receive compliantly the ministrations of the doctor. The doctor's role was to diagnose the cause of those symptoms, to develop a plan of care, and to direct the management of the care plan. In all of this, the patient remained, for the most part, the passive recipient of medical care.

This has been the traditional role of the patient for thousands of years: to be the passive recipient of whatever

---

3   It is both sad and ironic that the best research today suggests that very few open-heart surgeries reduced the risk of subsequent heart attacks or extended the life of the patient. "Is Heart Surgery Worth It?" Bloomberg Businessweek, July 18, 2005.

That Guy Nurse

care a physician, shaman, or medicine man declared necessary. And for all but the last half century or so, the physician was powerless against all but the most basic and minor maladies.

Now the medical world has changed. Medical science has evolved a means whereby, short of massive catastrophic trauma, few people in technologically developed countries need to die before attaining the full human life span of 90 or more years. It is the growing power of science that gives medicine victory over so many illnesses. And as science continued to gain strength and influence in medicine, the scope of medicine began to expand. In showing what worked to stop an illness, science began to reveal what caused the illness in the first place. Before long, medicine began acquiring the tools to achieve the "Holy Grail" of health care: prevention of disease.

The broad benefits of disease prevention are obvious. It is far more pleasant to avoid diseases—even treatable ones—especially when considering drug side effects, post-operative infections, and prolonged rehabilitation. Prevention can even save money: "A stitch in time saves nine." But that old adage contains a word that marks the divide between two worlds: time.

Time is the difference between treatment and prevention. Time is the divide between the world of repairing disease

The American Medical System:
Something Has Gone Terribly Wrong

and the world of maintaining health. Treatment cannot start until the problem is discovered. Prevention cannot succeed unless it begins before the problem. Treatment ends when the problem is solved or there are no further treatments. Prevention ends at the end of life.

At this point, you may well wonder what has just happened. You started reading about the old days versus the new and the doctor-patient relationship, and suddenly you're pondering time as the divide between two worlds. And when you consider that the author worked in philosophy before entering the real world, only to become a nurse in middle age, you might not be surprised if the train of thought got derailed a short way out of the station. Well, dear reader, you might be right most of the time. But in this case, there really is a connection. And, I would venture to say, this connection is the most important point of my book. Are you ready? Good. Because here it is.

The connection is you. You are the only thing connected to your health 100 per cent of the time. You and your health were born together, you've known each other practically your whole life, and you will die together. If your health is broken and you need someone to fix it, you spend a bit of your time with a doctor; when the treatment is done, the doctor is gone. But for the ongoing effort of maintaining your health over time, the only person you can count on to be there is you. From rolling up your sleeve for a vaccination to logging miles on a treadmill. From scheduling your next annual exam to scheduling time for exercise with your family. From bringing a list of questions for your doctor appointment to bringing a list of favorite healthy foods to the grocery store. The only one present through all these times is you.

That's what this book is all about. You are the only one who can control your health, and you, more than anyone else, live the consequences of your health choices. So you are responsible for maintaining your health. There's simply no other way! What I want for you and every American is to know how easily and well this can be done. But to do it easily and well, you will need to know some whys and wherefores about health and our medical system. And you will need a physician partner—someone you can trust and work well with, not just for those bits of time when you've lost your health, but for ongoing collaboration to maintain it. You will need a physician partnership that combines the trust and mutual commitment of the "good old days" with the disease-fighting and health-maintaining power of modern American medicine. You will need a doctor-patient relationship that is restored and revised for the 21st century (you'll find much more on this in Chapter 9).

This book is dedicated to helping people understand that the ultimate responsibility for health belongs

to each individual, not to the doctor and the medical system. It is dedicated to assist you, dear reader, first, to understand the foundations of lifelong health and, second, to understand the increasingly important role that you, the patient, must play in the medical system.

Finally, this book sets forth a vision for the future of medical care.[4] This vision entails changes in every area of medical practice: governmental (the role and function of the government), private (the roles of private insurance and of employers), practice (the roles of primary care doctors, of specialists, and of adjunct personnel such as nurses, nurse practitioners, and physician's assistants), and the new roles of the patient.

Note that in the title of this chapter, "The American Medical System: Something Has Gone Terribly Wrong," I do not refer to the American "health care" system. The United States does not have a health care system. The United States has never had a health care system. What it has is a medical system—a system designed to cure sickness and repair injury. And the system is very good at doing those things. But the truth of the matter is that health has very little to do with American medicine. In fact, it can reasonably be argued that we create no incentive for preventive care in the American

---

4   The details of this vision will be set forth in Part IV: A Vision for the Future of
    Medical Practice in the U.S.

That Guy Nurse

medical system—that is, doctors are virtually discouraged from keeping people healthy.

Think of your personal doctor. If your doctor is really good and spends time and energy listening to his patients and then teaching them and helping them take charge of their own health—thereby making all of his patients healthy—your doctor is going to be bankrupt. We do not pay doctors for having healthy patients. We pay them for curing illness and for fixing things that are broken.

Many businesses reward the employees who make the most of their product. They reward the employees who sell the most product. These are called "productivity rewards." But we do not reward doctors who produce the most healthy patients. We reward doctors who order the most tests or who perform the most surgeries. The system exists to make money, and there is very little money in good health.

Consider your local hospital. A serious outbreak of health in your hometown, and your hospital is in deep trouble. We do not reward hospitals for creating healthy communities.

Consider this, too. Most doctors work for large corporations. They no longer finish medical school and return to their hometowns and nail their shingle up on the front porch and go into practice. No. Today's physician is the employee of a large corporation worth millions, and often

The American Medical System:
Something Has Gone Terribly Wrong

sometimes billions, of dollars. It owns hospitals and clinics and surgery centers and urgent care centers. It employs tens of thousands of people. It exists for one primary reason: to make money. Each and every component of the system is expected to provide a return on investment.

The doctor is a component of the system. Patients have become, to a large degree, the raw material out of which the corporation generates profit. Even not-for-profit hospitals evaluate their success as well as the programs they offer primarily in terms of profit: of the degree to which their revenues exceed expenses. Emphasizing the shift to managing medical care using a business model is that today the doctor has become the "provider" and the patient has become the "consumer."

One of the most dramatic changes in the American medical system has been the demotion of the primary care doctor. The primary care doctor is the doctor the patient sees when entering the medical system. That's the doctor known in the mythology of the American medical system as the "family doctor." That's the doctor portrayed on early television and radio as a close family friend, full of wisdom, available at a moment's notice, and almost a member of the family from the cradle to the grave.

With the advent of modern corporate medicine, the

family doctor no longer exists. In his place is the "provider" who sees 25 to 30 "consumers" every day. In his place is the doctor whose primary job is to handle the most mundane and routine medical complaints and to refer everything else on to a specialist. In his place is the doctor whose relation to his patients is determined by the employer's decision to go with the lowest-cost provider of medical care. To make matters worse, that decision may be reviewed every year or two with the result that the consumer has a new doctor just that often.

While specialist salaries have been increasing rapidly over the past 20 years, the salaries of primary care physicians have been declining. Medical schools find it increasingly difficult to recruit students who want to go into primary care medicine. Primary care medicine is the bottom end of the totem pole. Between 1997 and 2005, the number of U.S. medical school graduates entering primary care medicine dropped by 50 percent. More and more the primary care doctor has become merely the gatekeeper who provides referrals to the specialists. And since the primary care physician's compensation is often determined by the number of patients seen, it becomes far easier and less costly (for the doctor) to send a patient to a specialist rather than to take the time to explain to the patient the nature of a problem and what the patient can do herself to deal with it and to prevent its recurrence.

The American Medical System:
Something Has Gone Terribly Wrong

This is a tragedy. **It is primary care medicine that can and must be the center of medical care.** It is the primary care doctor who must be given the opportunity to know his patients and to have his patients know him. It is the primary care doctor who can teach about issues of health and prevention. It is the primary care doctor who is the key to building a more healthy society and, perhaps, of equal importance, to controlling the destructive costs of medical care. In a time when the costs of medical care threaten patients, families, and society itself, it has been demonstrated that the degree to which primary care medicine is available, costs go down, patient satisfaction goes up, and outcomes improve.[5]

The American medical system is broken. Possibly it is broken beyond any reasonable hope of repair. And yes, we must each of us understand that system before it can change or before it can be, for us, a genuine health care system. I say a lot more about this in Part IV of this book, "A Vision for the Future of Medical Practice in the U.S."

By the way, we are constantly being told that America has the finest health care system in the world. We are told that people come from all over the world to participate in America's health care system. We are assured that we

---

5   Outside the Beltway, 1 November, 2007, Joyner, James, "Primary Care Physician Shortage," http://www.outsidethebeltway.com/archives/primary_care_physician_shortage/

certainly would not go to Canada for our medical care. In Canada, we are told, people are dying because they cannot receive medical care. In Canada, we are told, people have to wait a long time before receiving even basic medical care. In Canada, we are told, people leave in large numbers to come to the United States to receive medical care, which is both quick and better.

Let's consider some facts. In Canada, life expectancy is also greater than in the United States. In Canada, healthy life expectancy is greater than in the United States. In Canada, emergency care is equal to or better than the emergency care provided in the United States. In Canada (we are not usually informed of this) the per capita costs of medical care are substantially less than in the United States.

It has been suggested by some that saying these things is wrong, perhaps even unpatriotic. The facts, however, cannot be denied. The World Health Organization is the source of statistics through which we can compare medical care in the United States with medical care in all the other countries of the world.[6] The World Health Organization tells us that the United States ranks 27th among developed nations in life expectancy and that it ranks 37th among developed nations in healthy life expectancy. In 36 other countries, including

---

6   World Health Organization, see http://www.who.int/whosis/whostat/EN_WHS08_Full.pdf

The American Medical System:
Something Has Gone Terribly Wrong

some Third World countries, people stay healthy longer than they do in the United States.

To point this out is far from being unpatriotic. Given the tens of millions of Americans who have no access to medical insurance, government or private, and the tens of millions of others whose medical conditions are, in principle, preventable, this is a criticism intended to speak to those who can make a difference—a difference that will make America even greater than it is.[7]

Discouraging Statistics

But let's look at some facts. The United States currently spends two to three times more per capita for health care—that's two to three times more—than any other developed country on the planet. And yet the United States ranks 27th in longevity. In 26 other countries, people live longer on average than they do in the United States. Even more significantly, the United States ranks 37th in healthy longevity. There are 36 other countries, including some Third World countries, where people stay healthy longer than they do in the United States. The United States ranks close to last among developed nations in infant mortality. It ranks at the middle or below the middle in virtually every measure of medical outcomes.

---

7   Approximately 70 percent of all of the costs of medical care in the United States are for the treatment of what are common, in principle at least, preventable conditions.

And yet we spend two to three times more per person for medical care in the United States than anybody else.

These discouraging statistics are not solely to be attributed to the American health care system. The United States has a more ethnically diverse population and more poverty than other developed nations. Sadly, these facts contribute to these mediocre medical outcomes.

To put it most simply, there is very little money in **maintaining** health. Our medical system is not designed to promote health. It is designed to cure sickness and repair injury. It is designed to make a profit for its participants: hospitals, pharmaceutical companies, manufacturers of medical equipment, and insurance companies. Now there is nothing wrong with profit except when the goal of profit puts health and lives at risk. The dollars we spend for medical care are dollars spent almost entirely to cure and repair, not to promote health.

Primary care medicine, has, throughout most of the history of medicine, been exactly what its name says, "primary" medical care. But with the creation and growth of specialty medicine, primary care medicine has lost its preeminent position. Today the primary care physicians live at the bottom of the medical pecking order. Both in terms of prestige and income, the primary care physician

The American Medical System:
Something Has Gone Terribly Wrong

is at the bottom of the ladder. Fame and the wealth go to the specialties. But the specialties are designed to deal with patients who are either sick or injured. They have little or nothing to do with patients who are healthy and who hope to remain that way.

Out-of-Control Costs
Bill for Rick's Birth

May 29, 1942. Note the itemized costs of having a baby. My favorite line, "Circumcision, $3.00. You can't hardly get a good circumcision for $3.00 anymore".

Rick's mother had gone into the hospital, had a baby, and spent an entire week bonding, healing, resting, and learning. She went home with a bill for $67.25. You say, "Yes, but that was in 1942!" And yet, if nothing had changed from then until now except inflation, a woman should be able to enter a hospital, have a baby, spend an entire week, and go home with a bill for about $950.

I check at my hospital every so often. The last time was about six months ago. A young woman came in to have a baby on Monday morning. She was not allowed to come into the hospital until she was ready to deliver. I remember that when our daughter, Elizabeth, was born in 1967, Rosalie had called her doctor and told him her water had broken and that she was ready to go into labor at any time. She asked if it was okay if she just came in to the hospital. Her doctor responded that that was just fine. The young woman to whom I just referred called her doctor and told him that she was having contractions.

He asked, "How far apart are they?"

She responded, "Well, right now they are about 12 minutes apart."

He responded, "Call me back when they are five minutes apart."

The American Medical System:
Something Has Gone Terribly Wrong

She was not allowed to come into the hospital until she was truly ready to deliver. She came in on Monday morning, and had her baby, and on Tuesday afternoon, the mother and baby were discharged from the hospital with a bill for $5,000 that did not include the cost of the doctor. The system is out of control.

Let's acknowledge that lots of things have changed since 1942. The quality of the medical care that the mother and baby receive is far greater than it was then. We are far more able to handle difficulties in the birthing process. And today, given the growing presence of antibiotic-resistant bacteria, it is important to get the mother and the baby out of the hospital as soon as possible. Yet even with all of this, the increase in the cost of this care far exceeds the actual cost of the services provided, while the United States ranks last among all of the developed nations in infant mortality.

One reason for these out-of-control costs is that in the U.S., it has become very hard to die. Chapter 2 explores this disturbing situation in detail.

notes:

_____

_____

_____

_____

_____

_____

_____

_____

_____

_____

_____

_____

_____

_____

_____

The American Medical System:
Something Has Gone Terribly Wrong

It Has Become Very Hard to Die

It Has Become Very Hard to Die

Have I said this already? Yes. And I'll continue to say it, because understanding why it has become very hard to die is important to living long and dying healthy.

This lesson was impressed on me by one of my nursing mentors when I was orienting at the hospital, fresh out of nursing school. I was a 60-year-old man and my mentor was a 26-year-old woman. She was a skilled veteran nurse with five years of experience. At the nursing station on the cardiac floor, the patient call light would go on from one of my patients. I would answer and hear a voice saying, "I'm having chest pain." I would go ballistic. I just knew my patient was having a heart attack. This is what would happen:

I would dash down the hall to the room. Try to remember

the protocol for chest pain. Try to remember what the patient's chart said about prior history and reason for current admission. Check for diaphoresis (sweating) and other indications of pain or stress. Ask the patient to describe the location and intensity of the pain. If indicated, give a nitroglycerine pill under the tongue. Wait five minutes and reassess the symptoms. If no relief, give another nitro. Wait five minutes and reassess. A third nitro. If still no relief, call the cardiologist and report.

By the way, these incidents always seem to happen right in the middle of a shift, a time that is already very busy so that, in addition to standing by assessing the patient, I would also have to arrange for another nurse, also busy, to go to the room where a blood transfusion required checking every 15 minutes as well as to provide direction to my nursing assistant who wants to know what to do next. A doctor is waiting impatiently at the nursing station with new orders for her patient that she wants to give to me verbally. And on and on and on it goes.

Finally, observing my evident agitation and uncertainty, my mentor said to me one day, "John, cool it. You really have to work to kill a patient." It dawned on me that she was right. People are hard to kill. It's not like the movies. People have a stubborn resistance to dying. And modern medical science has made dying even more difficult

Death in the "Olden" Days

Until the middle of the 20th century, death, even in the United States, came faster than it does today. Medical science lacked the capacity to alter the natural trajectory of disease, infection, or trauma. Remember, life expectancy was 54. We died of myriad diseases unheard of today. A nasty cut could become infected and the infection could spread and kill. Simple trauma, a broken ankle, for instance, could generate a blood clot that, traveling into the lungs, could kill. Medical science had not yet invented medications that could prevent blood clots. Every city had a special hospital, a sanatorium, where patients with tuberculosis were sent for extended treatment and often to die. There may have been another hospital for children with scarlet fever. Contagious diseases sometimes meant that entire families were quarantined, with a sign prominently posted on the front of the house announcing that no one was allowed to enter or to leave.

The most striking part of death 50 years ago was how quickly and easily it came. That has been common throughout history, the natural state of things. Because of modern medical science, that situation has changed. Medical terminology refers to the period of illness that precedes death as "terminal morbidity." It refers to any medical condition, often a chronic condition, that eventually causes or substantially contributes to death. Examples of such conditions today are

It Has Become Very Hard to Die

heart disease, stroke, diabetes, and cancer. These, however, are examples of how we die today but not of how we died even half a century ago. As recently as half a century ago, the period of terminal morbidity was generally quite short, a matter of a few days, weeks, or maybe months, and people died from scarlet fever, mumps, chicken pox, tuberculosis, and polio. They died of traumas and infections that today are merely inconveniences. Mostly, though, they tended to die quickly, without the tens or hundreds of thousands of dollars of medications that did not even exist then and not after multiple surgeries through which a variety of organs were fixed, removed, or even replaced.

Today, however, often and with increasing frequency, it takes years to die. Patients are routinely said to have died after an extended "courageous battle" with whatever medical condition it was that took their life. Medical knowledge and skill have not just eliminated many of the causes of death experienced by our grandparents, they have allowed physicians to prolong life even when disease has stolen the patient's comfort, identity, and quality of life. Life is prolonged often to the end of the human life span.

In prior times, death just happened. It was very much a part of the natural order of things and it was almost fatalistically accepted. A story to illustrate:

Death Was No Big Deal

I had the weekend duty for hospice. My pager buzzed and I was directed to a home in a poor and rundown neighborhood of Green Bay. Arriving at the address, I knocked and let myself in per hospice protocol. In a darkened living room, an elderly lady sat in a rocking chair watching television. In the flickering light of the TV, I could make out the shape of a hospital bed in the dining room adjacent to the living room. In the bed was my patient. The lady in the chair nodded in that direction. As soon as I reached the bed, I realized that my patient was dead—he had been dead for some time, hours at least.

I went to the lady in the chair, his wife, and told her that her husband had died. In little more than a whisper, she said, "I know," and returned to watching the television. As I went about the business of preparing his body for delivery to the funeral director, called the doctor to have him pronounce the death, called the coroner to inform him, and called the mortuary to collect the body, her eyes never strayed from the TV. She answered my questions quietly and with no trace of emotion. Even when the mortuary staff arrived, placed the body in a body bag, loaded it onto a gurney, and moved out the front door, she never stopped watching the TV.

She may have been in a state of shock or denial, but I don't think so. And so it struck me, as it did on many other similar occasions, that I was in the presence of a person for whom, after a long marriage during which there had been sickness, joy, tragedy, merriment, births, and other deaths, there now came this death. This death had taken many months of surgery and medication and endless visits to the doctor or the hospital, but it had finally come. It was no big deal. It was just one more chapter in life's book and hardly worth missing an important part of the TV show for. This was not any lack of love or caring on the wife's part. Rather, it was just part of life to die. Her grieving process was long past.

It Has Become Very Hard to Die

> I thought of Tevye in the musical Fiddler on the Roof. He is thinking about love, and one day asks his wife if she loves him. Her outraged response: "Do I love you? Many years of washing your clothes, bearing and raising your children . . . and you ask, 'Do I love you?'"

In my hospice experience, I often encountered families whose love for the dying family member slowly turned into something else as the dying process extended for months and even years of repeated false alarms, each bringing the family together, sometimes from great distances, only to have them depart to await the next call that told them that the end was near. Love changed into something else as the primary caregiver(s) had put their lives on hold for months and even years as their time and attention was dominated by the needs of the dying person. Love changed into something else as the costs of care drained family resources even to the point of forcing bankruptcy

At some point in time death changed from a normal part of life to a medical event. Soon thereafter, a patient's death came to be seen as a failure. It marked either the failure of medical knowledge or the fact that someone had made a mistake. This notion of death signifying failure or defeat invaded both the medical world and society at large. As a nation, we came to think of death as something that could be put off indefinitely. Hawkeye Pierce, on TV's M*A*S*H*, while frantically attempting to restart a young soldier's heart, cries out, "Death is the enemy!" Our grandparents, however, saw it as stage of life, as natural as birth and eating and sleeping.

As medical knowledge and skill grew, and with it power over infections and traumas that throughout history had been fatal, it became the duty of the physician to "do everything." No possible medical intervention was to be spared to save life. Then, noble and inspiring as that may have been, the doctor could do little. The doctor would go to the patient's home with his black bag in which he carried virtually every available medication and instrument. If the patient couldn't be cured or repaired with what was in the bag, he either got better on his own or he died . . . and life expectancy was 54. The doctor could neither extend the period of terminal morbidity very far nor could he order medications or procedures that cost vast amounts of money.

Now medical science has given the physician the power to prolong life in ways unimaginable just a few decades ago, but, of course, this power has limits. The physician cannot restore all functions or cure all disease. As a result, we now have a world in which the pain and suffering associated with disease, trauma, and death are routinely extended over months, years, and even decades for millions who just a short time ago simply died. To add insult to all those injured and

It Has Become Very Hard to Die

suffering people, the prolonged, sophisticated treatments and medications have exponentially raised the financial costs of medicine. Note, too, that in all of these cases we are purchasing medical care, not health.

A Cautionary Tale

Just a few years ago, two dear family friends were bicycle riding in Door County, Wisconsin, a popular vacation area. Jane was 70 years old—a very active and fit 70. Suddenly, on a back road, her bicycle crashed and she lay on the pavement, unconscious. She'd had a cerebral aneurysm; a blood vessel in her brain had burst, and every time her heart beat, it did not circulate blood. Rather, it pumped the blood out into her skull. Quickly pressure built and she lost consciousness.

Bob, her husband, had just purchased a cell phone. He punched 911 and the rescue squad rushed to the scene. Jane was taken to Green Bay and placed on a medical helicopter for a flight to Madison. There surgeons carefully drilled a number of holes into her skull to drain the fluid and relieve the pressure on her brain. Her husband asked the surgeon, "Am I going home with Terri Schiavo?" For those of you who may not remember, Terri Schaivo suffered extensive brain damage, resulting in a persistent vegetative state and 15 years of institutionalization. In 1998, her husband petitioned the courts to have her feeding tube removed. Her parents sought an injunction, arguing that their daughter still was able to respond and to recognize things. Her husband's argument was that she had told him she'd never wanted to live that way. He did not have a durable power of attorney for health care through which his wishes would have been respected. As a result, a seven-year legal battle ensued before her feeding tube was removed. The president of the United States, the Congress and the Supreme Court were all involved before the matter was resolved.

In essence, Bob was asking if he was going to go home with his wife or with merely a vestigial remnant of her. The surgeon's answer was instructive. "She will survive." It was a classic answer from the American medical system.

For 10 days, Jane was stabilized. Her speech was slurred but she could speak. She did squeeze our hands when we requested it. Her eyes would follow us. But then she had a stroke. It took away movement in the entire right side of her body. It took away her ability to swallow. A feeding tube was surgically implanted through her abdomen and into her stomach. Bags of nutrients were hung at the side of the bed and pumped into her through the tube. As long as she lived, this would be how she took nutrients.

Jane was discharged to a nursing home in Green Bay for further evaluation and therapy. After about three weeks in

It Has Become Very Hard to Die

the nursing home, she suffered another aneurysm rupture. She was rushed to a nearby emergency room, where a shunt was placed at the base of her skull to drain fluid and pressure. In six days, the shunt was infected. Now there began a battle against infection. Again she was stabilized and returned to the nursing home. She was comatose. She could neither speak nor move.

The nursing home then called her husband to say that Medicare only paid for 30 days of rehabilitation and therapy. Jane had received that, but her condition was not improving. Therefore, the nursing home would subsequently have to bill Bob directly for Jane's care. That would be about $7,000 a month. At this point, Jane had not been at all responsive for a period of weeks. She did not speak. She could not respond to requests to squeeze your hand. She could not move.

Jane's daughter, Emily, had refused to accept that her mother was gone. She had organized Internet prayer groups all over the country to pray that God would send her mom back again. Finally, though, Emily accepted the fact that her mom was not going to return. Jane was admitted to hospice and brought home. The feeding tube was removed.

On the fourth night, I received a phone call asking if I would come and spend the night because Bob and Emily were exhausted and they did not want Jane to be left alone.

I sat beside her bed and held Jane's hand. A little before five in the morning, her heart began to race. I could not take a pulse on it. Her respirations increased to nearly 100 breaths a minute. I called Bob and Emily to come down. After half an hour, Jane stopped breathing.

Five months after her first ruptured aneurysm, Jane died. Her treatments cost approximately $1 million. I ask you to consider what incentive did anyone involved with this case— the corporation that owned and operated the hospitals and hired all the doctors and nurses or the corporation that owned and operated the various nursing homes—have to suggest at any point during this process that maybe it was time to stop. They made nearly $1 million in just five months from one patient.

I do not want to suggest that the doctors, nurses and other medical personnel involved in the care of Jane or any other patient would deliberately prolong life merely for the sake of money. I do want to insist that the medical system offers few incentives and fewer opportunities for those people to routinely stop, think, and challenge the wisdom of proceeding with a mission simply to prolong life.

It has become very hard to die.

So Who Is Paying for All This?

One other factor in the scenario of the medical extension of life expectancy has to do with cost. To an increasing degree, the costs of medicine are unrelated to questions of health. They are, on the contrary, spent to defer death. Unless one is involved in a situation so catastrophic that life is simply obliterated, the medical system will prolong life as far as science and technology can possibly reach. It makes little difference how much pain a patient may have to endure. It makes little difference how many thousands of dollars worth of medications come to line the walls of the kitchen or the bathroom. It makes little difference how many operations may be required. As Jane's doctor said, "She will survive."

So it is that the last consideration of all is cost. For those fortunate enough to have medical insurance, the costs of medical care are pretty well covered. But when the insurance reaches its limits (and this happens faster and faster today), it is required by law that the patient or the patient's family spend down whatever assets they may have until they reach a level of poverty, which entitles them to have medical care covered by Medicaid. The system will be paid. And, as mentioned above, as medical spending rises, it becomes clear that fewer and fewer dollars are going to buy health.

Is Anyone Minding the Cash Register?

With the growing technology of medical care and the growing capacity of medications to support essential life functions, we have entered into a time when the costs associated with medical care can and do escalate to a level that staggers the imagination. Through the institutions of Medicare and Medicaid, a rapidly increasing flow of dollars supports a growing volume of patients. An aging population, as well as a population of persons who are alive, having survived diseases and traumas that would, only a few decades ago, have been fatal, are rapidly increasing federal and state expenditures for medical care to the point that these costs are becoming dominant factors in the struggle to balance budgets while maintaining basic social needs for infrastructure, for safety, for community services, and for culture.

The following story illustrates both the power and expense of modern medicine:

While I was in nursing school, I worked part time as a nursing assistant. With just a few weeks of training, my job involved providing basic personal cares to homebound patients: feeding, bathing, dressing, and transferring them from bed to chair and back, that kind of thing.

One day I was assigned to a young man, Jim, who was

It Has Become Very Hard to Die

a quadriplegic. At age 19, he had gotten drunk and driven his car at high speed into a tree. His cervical spine (high in his neck) was broken, and he was completely paralyzed from the neck down. He could breathe without assistance except at night when he required a machine to breathe for him (a CPAP, a device worn over the face to force air into his lungs while he slept, since his paralysis did not allow him to breathe on his own while reclining). He could swallow only tiny bits of food and was always in danger of aspirating food into his lungs. From the neck down he had no capacity for voluntary control of any bodily function. Under the provisions of the Social Security Act, he was provided with a budget adequate for the employment of staff to be with him 24 hours each day, seven days a week. This allowed him to employ six people full and part time to attend him and to act as his arms and legs. Beyond this, medical staff was provided, and that is where I and other nurses and nursing assistants came in.

At seven o'clock every morning, one of the nursing assistants would arrive at Jim's house to begin the routine of getting him up. After waking Jim, the CPAP would be removed. Next a catheter bag affixed to his leg would be drained and stool that had accumulated would be digitally removed, since he was not capable of moving his own bowels. At this point, a registered nurse would arrive to give Jim his medications and to supervise the rest of the morning procedures.

A sling, a hammock-like affair, would be laid out on the bed and Jim would be rolled onto it. He was not capable of moving any part of his body other than his head, so moving a man who weighed in the neighborhood of 300 pounds was not an easy task. Once he was in the sling, it would be attached to an electric winch mounted to a track in the ceiling, and Jim would be carefully hoisted out of the bed. He would then be moved across the bedroom and into the bathroom, where the tub had been filled with warm water. He would be lowered into the tub and bathed. He would then be winched out of the tub and back to the bedroom, where he would be dressed and finally transferred into a wheelchair.

The wheelchair was itself a technological marvel. Jim could control it with a rod, one end of which he held in his teeth. With this rod, he could control the wheelchair to move forward and backward and to turn. At this point, the nurse would depart and the rest of the routine managed by the nursing assistant.

Jim would then move into the kitchen, where it would take about 30 minutes to feed him. He could only take sips of liquid and very small bites of soft food, and every bite or sip had to be fully ingested—and it had to be determined that he had not aspirated it into his lungs before the next bit or sip could be offered. At this point, one of his attendants would take over until evening when the entire morning procedure, with nurse and nursing assistant, would be repeated in reverse.

It Has Become Very Hard to Die

My acquaintance with Jim lasted only a few months. He was 26 at the time and devoted much of his time each day on a computer (operated with the tooth rod), provided to him as a Medicaid benefit, working with an organization whose mission was to increase the benefits available to quadriplegics. Jim and thousands, perhaps tens of thousands like him, live today only because of developments in medical technology and pharmacology that have occurred in the last few decades.

More Surgery? Why?

When I was a brand-new nurse who was still in the orientation phase of my job on the cardiac floor I was assigned a gentleman recovering from open-heart surgery. He was 83 years old and suffered from an advanced dementia, probably Alzheimer's. His dementia was so advanced that he responded only to pain stimuli and then only with inarticulate groans and grunts. He had lived for some time in a nursing home, and because he no longer was able to move voluntarily, his body had contracted into what can be best described as a fetal ball. His arms had contracted over his chest and his legs had pulled up tight until his feet were touching his buttocks.

While he was in the nursing home, it was discovered that he had a cancer in his penis. He was therefore sent to the hospital for a penectomy (the removal of penis). In the course of preparing him for that surgery, it was discovered that he had advanced heart disease. Therefore, he was prepared for and underwent open-heart surgery. I was to be his nurse during his recovery from that operation. Each day the dressing over his chest incision had to be replaced and the incision inspected for possible infection. This was not an easy task. It required that I have two nursing assistants standing on either side of the bed to pull his arms away from his chest and hold them while I changed the dressing. As soon as they released his arms they would snap forcefully back into their position across his chest. Through all of this there was no response. He recovered and subsequently sent back to surgery for the penectomy. Three days later I was "floated" to the med-surge floor where he again became my patient. His penis had been surgically removed and the scrotal sac sutured into his lower abdomen. A catheter had been inserted through his abdomen into his bladder to drain his urine.

I questioned the surgeon as to why these surgeries had been performed. He responded, "It was wrong. But if I hadn't done it, somebody else would have. It's what the family wanted."

It has become very hard to die.

An Inherent Conflict of Interest

Without dwelling on this topic, it is important to be clear that the primary goal of those institutions that comprise the American medical system—insurance companies, pharmaceutical companies, companies that manufacture medical instruments and appliances and diagnostic tools such as MRI scanners, the corporate entities that own and operate hospitals and clinics and that hire medical personnel—is profit. They exist to make money

This is not to suggest that there is anything wrong with the act of making money. Whatever the ethics or values of profit, however, this motivation creates a problem for the practice of medicine. Throughout all of history, and guided by the Hippocratic Oath, the motivation and goal for the doctor was the well-being of the patient. Today the doctor, with a few and rare exceptions, is employed by and answerable to corporate entities for whom patient well-being is at best a secondary interest.

There is thus an inherent conflict of interest in the American medical system. The doctor is trained in and ethically committed to placing the safety and well-being of the patient above and beyond any other considerations. At the same time, however, and to an increasing degree, the doctor's medical decisions are directed or even dictated by the other entities listed above. In all of this, the patient is as likely to be the victim as the beneficiary. The hows and whys of the situation will be made clear in later chapters. The bottom line, though, is that in the 21st century, the patient must assume an informed role and a level of involvement in the delivery of medical care unprecedented in history. More on this in Part II of this book: The Professional Patient.

A final illustration, if I may. As I stand giving one of my presentations, my face suddenly turns gray. I break out into a cold, clammy sweat. I clutch my chest, groan, and drop to the floor. I know precisely what's going to happen. In a nanosecond, a member of the audience will be on me like ugly on an ape. He will shake me and say, "Hey, are you okay?"

When I don't respond, whoever rushed up will check to see if I have a pulse . . . no pulse. He will check to see if I'm breathing . . . not breathing. He will shout out, "Call 911!" Then he will start CPR. Whoever rushed up will start chest compressions. Now, how do I know he will start chest compressions? Well, because he was the first person up here. The second person arriving, known as the "loser," will have to do mouth-to-mouth resuscitation. Within minutes, the rescue squad will arrive and they will inject my heart with a solution to dissolve the blood clot that caused my heart attack. I will not die.

If you want to die of a heart attack, you'd better go out in the deep woods and have it. Otherwise your chances of dying have become very small. Now, 40 years ago I would have been dead where I dropped. We did not have thousands of people trained in CPR. We did not have a 911 system. We did not have rescue squads. And if we had had them, they did not have the solution to dissolve the blood clot that caused my heart attack.

It Has Become Very Hard to Die

Of all of the vast amounts of money being spent for medical care in the United States today, the great majority are being spent for the treatment of illnesses and the repair of injuries. Virtually nothing is being spent to prevent sickness, injury, or very expensive chronic conditions that commonly accompany old age—especially old age achieved in spite of health-compromising lifestyles. More on this in Chapter 5, "Five Rules for Long-Term Health."

It has become very hard to die.

notes:

_____

_____

_____

_____

_____

_____

_____

You May Live 90 to 95 Years

In Chapter 2, I discussed how and why it has become very hard to die. Here I'll explain why, in all likelihood, you will live a very long time . . . perhaps 90 to 95 years.

Why 90 to 95 years? As was pointed out in Chapter 1, and it bears repeating, every living creature on this planet has a life span. The giant Sequoia has a lifespan of 2000 years or more. The Galapagos tortoise lives 175 to 200 years. Dogs tend to live 10 to 12 years, and cats get an extra year or two beyond that. Have you noticed that nobody keeps a fruit fly for a pet? You bring your little pet home from the store, build a little tiny house, and start teaching it tricks, and in 14 days it's dead. Fourteen days—that's the lifespan of a fruit fly.

The human lifespan is 90 to 95 years, a little more, or perhaps a little less. Notice that when somebody in your community has a 100th birthday or lives to 102, there is almost always going to be a story in the newspaper. Why?

Because that's news. What you must realize is that your being healthy has virtually nothing to do with your living to the full human lifespan. You're going to live that long because you will not be allowed to die.

Life Expectancy—A New Ballgame

Consider that it took the entire history of the human race until 1935 to get life expectancy up to 54 and now, in one lifetime, we've taken it to nearly 80. That's truly remarkable. It's even more remarkable when we realize that if we average our life expectancy together with that in the 26 countries

---

Actuarial Science and Me

Each day we live increases the odds that we will live longer. Let me illustrate. When I was 50 years old, if I decided that I wanted a life insurance policy, I would have called an agent. With virtually the speed of light he would be at my door. He would have a small book of actuarial tables and he would say, "Okay, you're a 50-year-old Caucasian male. Your life expectancy is 68." He would then write a life insurance policy figuring that if I died at the projected life expectancy of 68, the company could pay off the policy and still make a profit. If, however, I was 60 years old when I called that agent, his actuarial tables would have told him that I was now expected to live to 74. Again, premiums would be developed based on the policy having to pay off in 14 years. Now, in 2011, I am 76 and that same policy will require that the premiums be paid and the profit generated in about 7 years. That is, my life expectancy is now 83. And so it goes.

That Guy Nurse

where people live longer than we do and then average in all of the other nations on earth, a baby born today can expect to live just 46 years. I was born in 1935. That year life expectancy in the United States was 54. That's how long people lived on average, 54 years. Here in the United States our life expectancy is approaching 80.

Here's the kicker: Most Americans who have attained the age of 40 can now expect to live 90 to 95 years. You say, "But why? Life expectancy is only 80." The answer is that they have already survived the most dangerous parts of life. They didn't die in infancy, far and away the most dangerous part of the lifespan. They didn't die as children. They didn't die doing stupid teenage things. The chances are very small that anyone in their thirties and beyond will get sent off to fight a war somewhere. No, the odds are that great numbers of people alive today are going to live 90 to 95 years. Let's examine how and why.

It was only in the 1940s that antibiotics were discovered. Antibiotics are probably the greatest miracle in the history of medicine. With their discovery, almost overnight disease and infection ceased to be significant mortality factors for us. Hardly any American alive today is going to die of measles or mumps or chickenpox or diphtheria or polio or tuberculosis. Hardly anybody is going to die of scarlet fever or malaria or AIDS or other diseases that take the lives of hundreds of millions of people on this planet every year.

Only a few people will die of infection. Our grandparents and great-grandparents who experienced a bad cut on a hand or foot—a cut into which infectious organisms migrated and then migrated into the bloodstream and into the rest of the body—died. There was nothing the doctor could do about it. Today we are all immunized as infants, and literally thousands of medications have been created to control disease and infection. All over this planet, people die by the millions every year of diseases that none of us in the U.S. even think about.

Honesty requires mentioning two conditions that must be met in order to achieve living 90 to 95 years or longer.

Condition #1: The Element of Luck

First, you have to be a little lucky. There is bad luck in this world. A truck runs a stop sign and crushes a car and kills two people. That's bad luck. Lightning strikes a golfer on the ninth fairway. That's really bad luck. Infants are born with defective genes, and they either die quickly or suffer for a long time, and it's nobody's fault. Hurricanes, tornados, floods all strike and take lives. It is nobody's fault. It is just bad luck. The thing about luck, though, is that the chances that you will to die from bad luck are statistically almost 0.

The Flower Pot Incident

In early June 2007, I was moving a flower pot. It slipped and broke. I attempted to scoop up the potting soil and in the process, a shard of the pot cut my left ring finger. I washed the finger thoroughly and put bandage on it and then left town for two days to make presentations. By day two, I realized that the finger had become infected. As soon as I returned to Green Bay, I went to my doctor to have the finger checked. It was a staph infection, and I spent six days as an inpatient receiving IV antibiotics. The infection was cured. Had that same incident occurred 50 years ago, the odds are very good that I was a dead man.

Bad luck is the kind of thing that is shown on the television news and that we read about in the newspapers. The television shows us the car where two people died when a semi truck ran a stop sign. It doesn't show us the 14,000 cars that went through that intersection and nobody died. It shows us the dead golfer but not the 14 million golfers who golfed that day and did not get struck by lightning. Bad luck happens. You really can't do anything about it.

That said, though, it must be recognized that even with a fully responsible lifestyle, heeding all of the things we know about health and wellness, there are conditions that can threaten health and even directly cause death that are largely, if not completely, beyond the control of any individual. These fall in the category of the luck of the draw. Living near a factory that emits toxic pollutants, working in a plant

You May Live 90 to 95 Years

whose air is polluted from some manufacturing process, working in an office whose structural components emit toxic elements—these and many other environmental conditions threaten health and are to a large degree either unrecognized or unknowable.

There are many examples: the lead that was at one time used extensively in household paints and subsequently poisoned children; the asbestos used in construction that caused thousands of lung cancers; the toxic trans-fats used extensively in the production of pastries and fast foods and are now known to contribute heavily to heart disease. There are almost certainly more components of our environment that put us at risk but that are yet to be discovered. These things we cannot control or escape. There is also the bad luck of environmental disaster—the tornado, hurricane, flood, earthquake and all of the other ways in which life is destroyed but are nobody's fault.

All that said, the chances that you will die from bad luck are still almost 0.

Condition #2: Don't Do Anything Really Stupid

The second condition for living to 90 or 95 is this: you have to avoid doing anything really stupid. Maybe you've heard of the Darwin Awards? These are awards given to people who, because they've done something terribly stupid, have helped to empty out the shallow end of the gene pool. One of my favorites concerns a college student who joined a group of his friends on the roof of their high-rise dormitory to have a competition. The competition was to see who could spit the furthest over the edge of the roof. This brilliant student decided that he could spit the furthest if he backed up all the way across the roof and got a running start. You can guess what happened. He ran so fast before he spit, he threw himself off the edge of the roof.

A further award came about when on 2 February 2008 in New York state, a 50-year-old man was bird hunting with his buddies and his faithful canine companion. They stopped for a smoke, and his dog found a deer leg bone!

The man tried to take the bone away, but like any right-thinking dog, the animal would not relinquish its treasure. He stayed just out of reach. Frustrated with this blatant show of disobedience, the man grabbed his loaded shotgun by the muzzle and began wielding it like a club. Each time he swung it, the dog dodged.

Suddenly the "club" struck the ground and fired, shooting the man in the abdomen. He was airlifted to a nearby hospital, where he died from his injuries. He did remain conscious long enough to confirm this account to police; otherwise his poor friends might now be under suspicion!

At least he didn't hit the dog.[1]

Yes, people die from being stupid.

Say you have a burned-out light bulb high in your ceiling. You could go down to the basement and get a stepladder and drag it upstairs and set it up and climb the ladder and change the bulb. But that's not what you do, is it? No, you get a tippy little kitchen stool and stand it on top of the counter and climb up on top of it to reach the bulb. And when you fall and wake up in the emergency room, you clap your forehead and say, "Darn, that was a stupid thing to do!"

Yes, we all do stupid things. But the chances that we will die from being stupid are very small. We break things, bruise things, cut things, and scrape things, but we rarely die from being stupid. You will, in all likelihood, live a long time. You will not be allowed to die. So it is up to you to do everything possible to ensure that your long life will be lived in good health.

---

1   www.Darwinawards.com

A Favorite Stupid Story

It happened in Green Bay about five years ago in early March. The temperature was about 34 degrees and it was snowing, the type of heavy, wet snow that comes in the early spring. A guy in Green Bay was so concerned that the weight of all that snow on his new roof was going to damage it that he got a stepladder and went up on the roof to shovel off the snow. So far so good. It turns out that this fella was three fries short of a Happy Meal. His wheel was turning but the hamster had died. He completely ignored the fact that he had put the foot of the stepladder on a patch of ice on his concrete patio. When he was done shoveling, he stepped on the ladder to come down. The foot of the ladder slid away from the house, and he crashed down 12 feet and landed on the ladder on the concrete and . . . I broke my left arm.

The Fantasy of My Own Death

I've been around death for a long time. On the cardiac floor of the hospital, not every surgery succeeds. We lose patients. In hospice homes, everybody dies. Some years ago, faced with so much death, I began to think about my own death and how I want to die. Slowly, I've developed a fantasy of my own death. I want to be 94, and if all goes well, one day in my 94th year—I certainly can't know what day it will be—but on that day, if all goes exactly right . . . I will be shot by a jealous husband. That's my fantasy. Men do have fantasies. My wife, Rosalie, isn't too happy about this fantasy, but that's a different story.

So that's a fantasy. How do I really want to die? I would like to be 94 (and I'll take a hundred if I can get it). One day in my 94th year, when I wake up in the morning and toss the covers off the bed, my very first thought will be, "I feel good!" I think this every morning. It is wonderful to be able to wake up and think, "I feel good."

I will get out of bed. My body will be terribly unhappy with me. My body is 94 years old. It is stiff, sore, and achy. It wants to stay in bed. I will force it out of bed, though, and make it go through all of my morning stretching exercises to get loosened up and ready to go. I will have some breakfast. Then I will go out into the world to spend the day doing whatever it is I want to do. I'm pretty certain I will still be a nurse. This was a great decision for me, and I have no intention of retiring.

In addition, for most of my life, I have enjoyed long-distance bicycle riding. Forty years ago when my friends and I wanted to do a ride, the big deal was to do a "century". You would get on your bikes on a Saturday morning and you would ride 100 miles. Destination made no difference. The whole point is to ride 100 miles. You would come home at the end of the day tired and butt sore, but you did accomplish the century. I have to admit that I don't do centuries anymore. I'm good for 60-to-80 mile days but not for centuries. And on that fateful day when I'm 94, I figure maybe 12 miles will be a good bike ride.

Whatever I do, though, I'm coming home that night to have some supper, read a chapter or two, watch some TV, and go to bed . . . and people will say, "Was that ever something! He lived every day of his life right up until the very end, and then he died so peacefully in his sleep." But, you see, that's the way it's supposed to be—*that's exactly the way it's supposed to be.*

I did not die after years or decades of increasing pain and disability. I did not die after endless surgeries and with thousands of dollars worth of medications lining the walls of the kitchen and the bathroom. I did not die being cared for by my children who, in their 60s, were dreaming of their own retirement adventures but instead they're taking care of me. I did not die in some institution being fed pureed food three times a day by an attendant who then has to wheel me into the bathroom to change my adult diaper because I'm incontinent. I did not die so overmedicated that I did not know who I was or where I was. I died after a day on the bike.

And you say, "You died?"

And I say, "Yes."

"But why did you die?"

"I died because I got old."

The Way It Should Be

If you're at all like me, you probably grew up thinking that you have to die from something. You grew up thinking that death is some sort of a medical event, and if only we had more medical knowledge or somebody hadn't made a mistake, well, then maybe . . . But all of us will die. That's a given. And if all goes just the way it should, we will die after 90 to 95 years, a little less or a little more, and we will die in relative peace after a very short time during which we are not fundamentally in control of our lives. That's the way it should be. That's exactly the way it should be.

We still do not know very much about growing old. If you doubt that, go online to Google or some other search engine and type in the words "theories of aging." You will discover how many different theories of how and why we age are currently being researched. And that shouldn't seem so strange.

Consider this: It is 1938, I am a child, and I am sick. My mother calls the family doctor. She says, "Doctor, John is sick. He has a fever. He's throwing up. He's chilled. He has a rash. What should I do?" And what does the doctor say? He says, "I'll be right over." Up until the 1950s, if you needed a doctor, chances were the doctor came to your house. And why did the doctor come to your house? The doctor had a black bag. And in that black bag the doctor carried virtually every medication and every medical instrument available. If you could not be cured with what was in the black bag, you got better on your own or you died.

We died by the tens of thousands of measles and mumps and chickenpox and diphtheria and scarlet fever and polio and many, many other diseases, and there was nothing the medical profession could do about it. We died of broken ankles that sent blood clots migrating into our lungs because medicine had not yet developed blood thinners. **We died of accidents that, today, might not even have us go to the local urgent care clinic.**

In the days when medical professionals were not capable of keeping us alive in infancy and childhood or after accidents and infections, nobody in medicine was thinking, "What do we have to do if we want to stay healthy in our 50s and 60s and 70s and 80s and 90s?" Back then there was very little that they could do. There were very few medications. There were very few available surgeries, and those that were available were dangerous.

But then medicine got good. It has gotten very good at keeping us alive. But when all is said and done, it's up to each and every one of us to stay healthy.

For some these facts provide the foundations for a

fatalistic view of life. "When it is your time, you die. There's not much you can do about that." This view, however, is simple and shortsighted. Even without guarantees, we can maximize our odds, and I know of very few fatalists who do not practice, to some degree, the habits of everyday safety.

The Unknown and the Unknowable

After one of my talks, I was approached by a man who expressed concern about my emphasis on individuals being responsible for their own health. His mother died at age 62 of breast cancer. She had no family history of cancer. She did not smoke. She had regular mammograms. It would appear that she had done nothing to put herself at risk, and yet she contracted and died from breast cancer discovered when she had a mammogram. He felt that life was simply a crap shoot.

I can imagine ways in which her demise might have been prevented. I do not know how frequently she had mammograms. I do not know if the cost of mammograms was reimbursed by her insurance or if she even had insurance. I do not know how competent her radiologist may have been in reading mammograms. I do know, though, that there is, in every event in life, some dimension of the unknown and the unknowable. *There is, as we said earlier, always some element of luck in our lives.*

That Guy Nurse

The fundamental fact that must be accepted is that life carries no guarantees of fairness. What we can do is to maximize the odds in our favor. We cannot control our genetic inheritance, our age, or our gender. We can control, to a far greater degree than has been heretofore thought possible, those life circumstances that increase our odds of a long and healthy life. So you can reasonably expect to live to 90 to 95 years. That's no longer a challenge. The challenge each of us faces is to come to the end of life in reasonably good health. Stay tuned for more on this.

notes:

_____

_____

_____

_____

_____

_____

_____

_____

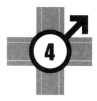

As We Age: Sagging and Bagging

Before we talk about the requirements for staying healthy for the full life span—trust me, we'll get there soon, in the next chapter—I want to briefly discuss the things that happen as we age. For unless we understand the changes that occur with aging, we cannot possibly understand the things we need to do to prepare for and to deal with those changes. We cannot stop the aging process, but we can, to a far greater degree than has ever been thought possible, deal with these aging changes in such a way that they do not take away our lives or our quality of life.

To kick off this discussion, here's a typical scene from one of my presentations:

She Thinks I Look Older Than Dirt, But She's Too Polite to Say So

An audience member is selected and I ask her name. Then

I ask her, "Jean, have you ever met me before?"

"No."

"So, the first time you ever saw me was when I was introduced, is that right?"

"Yes."

"Now, Jean, I've done this so many times that I've become something like a mind reader. I can pretty well tell exactly what you thought when you first saw me. The very first thought in your mind was, 'Oh my gosh, that is the best looking man I have ever seen!' Now, Jean, that's okay. I've carried this problem around with me almost all of my life, and I've come to accept it. But Jean, as you saw me and had that thought, you were probably immediately aware that there's no possible way that I could be 15 years old. Is that correct?"

Silence.

"Jean, look at me and tell me how you can tell that I'm not 15 years old."

At this point, and usually with lots of laughter from the audience, Jean struggles. I usually suggest to the audience, "She thinks I look older than dirt, but she's too polite to say so." Eventually Jean will suggest that I'm bald. I respond that I have a full head of hair but that it's cut very short. She suggests that my eyebrows are gray. I point out that any 15-year-old could dye his eyebrows gray. This conversation goes on for some time, but eventually Jean will point out that my skin has wrinkles.

"Yes, my skin is saggy and baggy and wrinkly, and that's only what you can see. That's all right, ladies and gentlemen, women have fantasies, too."

Cosmetic Changes and Those that Affect Health

As we age many things change. Some people grow bald. Some grow gray. Ear lobes elongate and nose tips droop. Most of the changes that occur with aging are cosmetic and not terribly serious. However, every tissue in our bodies, and the skin is only one of many tissues that make up our bodies, will become saggy and baggy as we grow old. Most of my face hangs under my chin. What used to be a great chest is now called a waist. But I am old, and everything has gotten saggy and baggy.

If I happen to be speaking to an audience with a number of young people, I will ask one of them to pinch the skin on the back of their hand lift it up and let it go. That young skin will immediately snap back into place. Then I lift up the skin on the back of my hand. When I let it go, it doesn't snap back. It just stands up just the way it was when I let go. Often the people who are observing this will respond with "Yuck."

Not all of the changes that occur with aging are significant in relation to the issue of good health. Many mean nothing, and others are primarily of cosmetic interest but have no bearing on the questions of health except possibly for the health of our egos. In this category, we might place the lengthening of the ear lobes and the drooping of the tip of the nose. Balding and the graying of the hair are typical but not matters of genuine concern where health is the object. Young men are usually not aware that one day they will grow long black hairs in their ears and noses.

In our 50s, the shape of the eye begins to change, and those of us who have been 20/20 all our lives now find we either have to hold the newspaper at arm's length or get glasses. The ability to hear the higher pitches goes away, and the truly old may lose the ability to understand high-pitched voices. Sexually it may become more difficult for males to sustain erections and for women to achieve adequate genital lubrication prior to intercourse. Toenails tend to thicken, and the skin becomes thinner and more susceptible to damage. The loss of melatonin in the skin may lead to the emergence of "age spots" on the backs of the hands or face. These and many other age-related changes occur—and let's face it, they're not fun—but they do not, by themselves, affect health.

We know how vital exercise is for the body to retain its maximum functioning. But we are also becoming aware that the mind demands to be exercised as well. As people retire from active engagement with the world, involved in their jobs and in other community activities, the mind is no longer challenged and, like the body without exercise, it may begin to fail. Good mental exercise is achieved with reading, doing puzzles, and being actively engaged in the world where decisions have to be made and in which those decisions make a difference.[1] Doing crosswords or Sudoko puzzles is great mental exercise. Many board games, such as Monopoly, provide mental challenge and demand focused attention. Chess and even checkers can provide good mental exercise. Almost any activity that requires that we use our minds to solve puzzles and that challenges and focuses our attention may help slow the aging process.

Other changes that occur with aging, however, have a direct and vital bearing on the ability of the body and mind to remain functional. Chief among these changes is the loss of tone and mass in the muscular system. To one degree or another, all of the tissues in the body, the skin being the

---

1   There is little empirical evidence to support the contention that mental exercise slows the process of mental aging. Yet most researchers in this area suggest that it will be better to act as if the hypothesis were true pending the availability of results from long-term scientific research.

As We Age: Sagging and Bagging

most obvious, loose the tight elasticity that they had when we were young. To a degree, the loss of tissue elasticity can be compensated for through plastic surgery and with the application of anti-wrinkle creams and lotions. But these processes are in no way "anti-aging". They merely alter the superficial and outward appearance of aging. "Tummy tucks" and surgery for sagging eyelids, facelifts, and other surgical gimmicks may serve the needs of the ego for a while, but they in no way alter the progress of the aging process.

In addition, up and down our spines, between each of the vertebrae that make up our spines, there are shock-absorbing discs. When you we get really old, these discs begin to shrink and dry up, and we lose altitude. We get short. You've all had the experience of driving down the highway and coming up behind another car. It's usually a Buick. And there's no driver. "Oh my gosh! There's is no driver in that car!" you think. And then you pass the car and see a little old person trying to see out over the dashboard. That person used to be three to four inches taller, but he grew old and his spine collapsed.

Starting in our 40s, we begin to lose muscle mass. Every year some portion of our muscle mass simply goes away. When life expectancy was 54 or even 60, that made very little difference. But remember, we are probably going to live 90 to 95 years or longer. We're going to get tiny. How tiny? Visit any nursing home and select any resident there. Get their permission and then go into their room. Almost always you will find photographs taken 50 or 60 years ago when the resident was young. And you can compare the person in the photograph to the person in the bed or the wheelchair and see what 50 or 60 years of losing muscle mass can do.

As we age, our nutritional needs also change. They change in terms of the number of calories required to maintain a healthy weight, and they change in terms of the foods required for health. For example, as muscle mass diminishes with age, so do our caloric requirements. It is a sad and sobering thought, but if our weight remains constant as we get older, it is only because we are replacing muscle with fat.

And therein lies the beginnings of a tragic story told millions of times over. When I was born and people older than I were born and life expectancy was 54 or even less, nobody in medicine was thinking about what had to be done to stay healthy through one's 50s and 60s and 70s and 80s and 90s. Then medicine medical science got good, and we launched an entire population into living a long, long time with hardly any understanding of what is required in order to stay healthy for all of that time.

As life expectancy in the United States began to grow rapidly in the 1950s, we were confronted with a growing number of people whose bodies were crippled, who needed to consume more and more of the growing supply of new and different drugs, who needed more and more surgery to repair parts that were broken or that no longer worked, and who became utterly dependent on being supported by others in the performance of the most basic functions of life.

It was natural—indeed inevitable—that we would think this situation developed simply because people were growing older and that these changes were simply a function of age. Nothing could be further from the truth. The application of medical knowledge was helping people live longer. But at the same time, the American diet was evolving into the massively high fat and high sugar diet of today. Many, if not most, of the foods we eat today did not exist 60 years ago, especially processed foods, which some argue are not foods at all.[2] Manufactured products were increasingly sold on the basis that they were "labor saving". We grew older, and as machines took over the work of life, we became a sedentary society. And as we have now learned, consuming a high-fat, high-sugar diet while living a sedentary life is ultimately destructive of health.

It has only been in the last few decades that there has been serious research into how and why we age. It is interesting to go online and to Google the topic "theories of aging." There are many such theories, each being researched as scientists

2   *In Defense of Food.* Michael Pollan. Penguin Press. New York. 2008.

That Guy Nurse

try to understand what is happening to people as they move into their 70s, 80s, 90s and beyond. So we age and are only now beginning to understand how and why and what we can do about it.

At the same time, we have become an "ageist" society. We make jokes about having "senior moments". We make jokes about seniors and sex. We believe, without thinking about it too much, that growing old inevitably entails a loss of mental function as well as of physical capacity. We believe

---

A Recreational Contrast

Recently a friend and I decided to drive down to Madison, Wisconsin, to kayak the lakes of Madison. We are sea kayakers. Our boats are 17 feet long and designed to go long distances on flat water. We launched on Lake Mendota and paddled the shoreline to the locks on the Yahara River. We paddled down the river and then across Lake Monona and into Lake Waubesa. We then returned by the same route. We were on the water for about six hours. During the entire trip, we did not see another kayak, canoe, or rowboat.

We were, though, surrounded by power boats. There were jet skis. There were outboards. There were inboards/outboards. There were cabin cruisers. Literally hundreds of powerboats threw up crosscurrents of wakes that sometimes threatened to overturn our kayaks. The great majority of those boats were carrying young people, people in their 20s and 30s and 40s. My friend who, like me is in his 70s and is a recently retired cardiologist, commented, "What's wrong with this picture?"

As We Age: Sagging and Bagging

that with age comes disease and a crippling of the body. We are, in other words, prejudiced with respect to growing old. And because we believe these things about growing old, we accept them as being in some sense inevitable. We then become the victims of our own prejudice. We believe these things and then become fatalists as we accept them.

It is important to understand that although the body and the mind change as the years roll by, these changes need not be destructive of our quality of life. They are just changes, and, like all other changes, they bring us challenges as well as opportunities. But only in understanding the changes that are occurring and that will occur can we even begin to understand the decisions that we have to make if we wish to come to the end of life experiencing the joy of fundamentally good health.

It's All About Adapting

Life, from birth to death, is all about adaptation. We are constantly adapting ourselves to our environment. Unless we do so, we cannot survive. We feel hunger and so we eat. We feel cold and so we dress warmly. We feel thirst and so we drink. We feel bored and so we choose an activity that excites us. Many adaptations are done without conscious thought. In the autumn, as temperatures drop and the days grow short, many birds depart the northern climes and fly south. The birds are not sitting on a fence post or a power line thinking, "My gosh, it's getting cold and the days are getting short. We'd better start heading south." No, we refer to their behavior as "instinctual." The birds are genetically hard wired to perform a certain behavior under certain conditions.

Likewise, we human beings are genetically hard wired to a variety of behaviors that we perform without conscious thought. For example, when we get cold, we shiver. The shivering generates heat to offset the cold. But we do not think to ourselves, "Boy, I'm getting cold. I think I had better start shivering." When exposed to cold temperatures that could be threatening to life, our bodies shut down circulation to our feet and hands and ears. They increase circulation to the internal organs, those organs vital for life. And this adaptation happens without conscious thought.

Being human means that we can also think. We can engage in problem-solving behavior. Thinking and reasoning are tools we have to increase our ability to adapt and thereby to survive. For example, we live in a world in which most people no longer have to engage in daily hard work in order to have the food they need or shelter from the weather. We can spend entire careers sitting at computer terminals or riding a forklift in the factory. We mostly don't walk to the store for groceries. We get into our cars, turn on the air conditioning, and circle the parking lot at the supermarket to find a parking place as close as possible. Being busy and seeking convenience, we eat fast foods that have little or no nutritional value. Because we do not engage in regular exercise at work or for recreation, we build up stress. Stress that is not relieved through exercise eventually weakens and then destroys our auto-immune system. Then we become vulnerable to some very bad things.

Our bodies are constantly changing, and with each change, the adaptations that we must make to remain healthy also change. Our bodies and our minds demand exercise and a proper diet. They demand sleep. Our eyes change and we adapt with glasses. Our hearing changes and we adapt with hearing aids. In hundreds of ways, our bodies and our minds undergo change as we age. As they change, the requirements of adaptation change. Maintaining life long health thus requires that we understand what is happening and how we need to do to adapt.

Finally, medical science is turning to the task of understanding the process of aging and the needs of the aging person to adapt in new and different ways. Unfortunately, however (as has been explained in Chapter 1), the American medical system has made it difficult if not impossible for primary care doctors to fulfill their role as teachers. The result is that we are a nation of people who are medically illiterate. Until the system changes and restores to the primary care doctor the time and the opportunity to be a teacher (as will be discussed in Part II, The Professional Patient), it remains the responsibility of each of us to learn what we can to understand the aging process. In the next chapter, we will begin to explore the foundations of lifelong health.

notes:

_____

_____

_____

_____

_____

_____

_____

_____

As We Age: Sagging and Bagging

The Five Rules for Long-Term Health

Okay! We're finally at Chapter 5 (if you didn't skip ahead—and if you did, that's just fine). This is the clear, tailor-it-for-yourself, how-to portion of my message. I'm about to share with you what I think of as the five foundational elements—the Five Rules—for long-term health. The details will change over time as we learn more about aging and health. The foundations are, though, pretty secure. Here we go.

Rule #1: Exercise

The essential, nonnegotiable foundation of long-term health is . . . ta da! Exercise! I'm not talking here about trying for six-pack abs and buns of steel. I have those and I won't live a day longer because of it. But know this: should you choose to stay healthy as long as you will be alive, you must engage in regular exercise.

Let me digress for a moment and focus on the word "choose." Please understand, health is a choice! It's very easy to take health for granted because our bodies have been so wonderfully designed that most of them are good for 50 or 60 years in good health without our doing anything at all. Think of it as a health account.

Your Health Account

The day you were born there was set aside for you a bank account called the "health account." It was big. It was massive. It was so big that you could write checks on it every day, week, month, and year you lived and there was always a balance left. However, for most of us, after 50 or 60 years, the health account is nearly empty. We are almost "healthrupt". Unless we are prepared to make regular deposits back into that account, we will one day be totally "healthrupt".

The rule is this: if you choose to stay healthy for as long as you will be alive, you must exercise a minimum of three to five times each week. Each exercise session must last for a minimum of 20 to 30 minutes. During that entire time, your heart rate must be raised to a rate appropriate to your age. The formula for determining that heart rate can be found in the Resources section at the end of this book.

Now, I did not make up the rules. But the rules are

absolute and clear. Unless you commit to a program of regular, vigorous exercise a minimum of three to five times each week—with your heart rate raised to an appropriate level for each minute of that exercise—it is as sure as that God ever made little green apples that your heart will fail, and that's when you come into the American medical system for real.

The heart is a muscle. As we age, it loses some of its mass, and like every other tissue in our bodies, it becomes flabby. When we were young, on a summer afternoon, running around and playing, our hearts could easily achieve rates of 170 or 180 beats a minute. My heart is now as flabby as my face. I try to work out every day for as much as an hour, but my heart long ago gave up any hope of beating 170 or 180 times a minute. I get a good quality workout at 115 to 120 beats a minute.

And on that fateful day when I am 94 years old and I see the jealous husband raising his gun at me (remember my fantasy from Chapter 3?) and I am in a state of almost hysterical panic, my heart will go only about 90 beats a minute.[1] And finally the time will come when my heart cannot beat hard

---

[1] To illustrate how your heart rate changes with age try this: Get a watch with a sweep second hand. Place it where you can see the second hand. Now clap your hand three times every second, or 30 times every ten seconds. That is the rate of a young heart. Next, clap twice every second, or 20 times every ten seconds. This is the rate of a heart 70 years old. Finally, clap three times every two seconds. Now you have the rate of a 90-year-old heart.

The Five Rules for Long-Term Health

If You Don't Exercise:
A [Depressing] Peek into the Future

As your heart begins to fail, the first thing your doctor will do is to write you a prescription for a medication, Digoxin, to strengthen and regulate your heartbeat. Every time your heart beats, the medication kicks in and your weakened heart gets some strength back. But nothing stops the aging process, and even on the medication, the heart becomes weaker until one day you discover that your feet are beginning to swell. Your heart is no longer strong enough to keep the kidneys operating, and you retain fluids. Gravity draws the fluids to the lowest part of your body, your feet. Your feet begin to fill with fluid. This is called "edema." As fluid accumulates, the heart has to work even harder. Since it is already weakened, its failure accelerates.

Now your doctor orders another medication, Lasix. You take one or two Lasix pills each day, and you pee like a racehorse. You dump off the accumulating fluid. This, too, is good. However, the aging process moves on, and before long, you have maxed out on Digoxin and you've maxed out on Lasix and then slowly, inexorably, you will drown in your own fluids. That's called "congestive heart failure." Millions of Americans have congestive heart failure. Without regular vigorous exercise, this outcome is almost certain.

enough or fast enough to keep itself going . . . and it will quietly and peacefully stop. And that's the way it's supposed to be. That is exactly the way it's supposed to be.

But without regular, vigorous exercise, your heart does not stand the chance of a snowball in hell of making it.

That Guy Nurse

The Magic Bullet

Exercise has so many other benefits. It's almost like the fabled magic bullet that can cure everything. The single most prescribed medications in the United States today are anti-depressant and anti-anxiety medications. Yet we know that approximately 70 percent of those people who suffer such acute episodes of anxiety and depression that their doctor writes them a prescription for Prozac (or Wellbutrin or Zoloft) would not need those medications if they exercised.[2]

Exercise is also an effective means for achieving weight control. And for reasons not fully understood, it reduces one's risk of a number of cancers.[3] Finally, there are benefits of exercise still to be discovered.

When I give my talks and get to this section on exercise, I have yet to have somebody approach me to say that I don't know what I'm talking about—that the secret to long healthy life is to go home each night, watch a lot of television and drink beer. No. What I hear from people is something like this: "I know I should exercise. I know it's good for me. The big problem is I just don't have the...time." Yes. It's an individual decision, to exercise or not. But it is absolutely certain that unless a person chooses to make the time to exercise, his body will eventually destroy itself. Exercise is

2   http://www.mayoclinic.com/health/depression-and-exercise/MH00043
3   http://cancer.about.com/od/causes/tp/exercise.htm

The Five Rules for Long-Term Health

My Summers on the Farm

When I was a child, my parents sent me to the family farm in central Wisconsin. This was in the 1940s, and there was no electricity there. Each day began about five in the morning with milking 35 cows by hand. Following the milking, the barn had to be cleaned with a broom and a shovel; then we pitched fresh hay down from the mow and laid in each stanchion area. After breakfast, we would hitch up the horses and I would follow the them around the fields all morning picking up rocks. We grew great rocks on that farm.

At noon, more often than not, grandma would announce that the garden needed to be weeded. This was not a hobby garden. This was the garden where we had to raise most of the food that we lived on all year long, with a little extra to take into town on the weekends. And grandma never gave me an 8-horsepower Roto-tiller to weed the garden with. She would hand me a hoe and I would spend the afternoon pulling weeds.

On the worst days, she would announce that we were going to have chicken for supper. You can guess who had to go out and chase a chicken, catch a chicken, kill a chicken, clean a chicken, and then chop and carry the wood to cook the chicken with after he had pumped and carried the water to cook the chicken in. We didn't have Kentucky Fried Chicken or McDonald's. We didn't live near a supermarket with acres of meats and grains and fruits and vegetables from all over the world every season of the year. We had what we raised by the sweat of our brows. And I didn't work as hard as grandma or grandpa.

one of the very best ways to make deposits into the health account.

There is an amazing irony in this. Our grandparents and great grandparents generally had to work their butts off every day just in order to survive. On the farm, in a factory, or at home, every day involved hard physical labor.

When I was a boy, one of the great thrills on a summer afternoon was when the truck from the telephone company or the electric company would come into our neighborhood. We kids knew we were in for a show. We would crowd around the truck. The door would open and a man would step out. To us, he was like the fabled Paul Bunyan. We would watch as he strapped a massive and very heavy tool belt around his waist. He strapped hooks to his feet and legs. He walked over to the nearest utility pole, threw a heavy leather safety belt around the pole, and strapped the safety belt to his tool belt. Then he slowly dug his hooks into the pole, threw his safety belt up to go higher, dug in, and climbed higher. It was an amazing sight!

Today, though, the romance has gone out of it. The truck drives into the neighborhood. The man gets out and climbs into a plastic bucket at the back of the truck. He pulls a tiny handle and the bucket slowly rises up into the sky, where the man does whatever it is he supposed to do. It ain't the same, but it is a mark of our time that by and large we no longer have to work. And without work and exercise, it is in the very nature of things that our bodies will destroy themselves.

Exercise is the essential foundation for staying healthy as long as you will live. And that's a fact.

One More Benefit of Exercise: the Importance of Stretching[4]

An important—some would say vital—activity for those who choose health is stretching. With aging, muscles not only lose mass, they contract; they get shorter. As muscles contract, particularly those in the legs, there is an increased loss of balance and corresponding increase in the danger of falling, Fifty percent of people over 75 will either die or be forced to enter institutional care because of falls. Stretching, properly done, should always be part of our exercise routine. Here again, your primary care doctor can be an excellent resource in determining how to stretch for maximum benefit.

Rule #2: Fuel the Machine

The average American consumes a diet consisting of 35 to even 70 percent fat. Rule #2 is that the diet should consist of no more than 25 percent fat, and that most of that 25

---

4   http://www.mayoclinic.com/health/stretching/HQ01447

That Guy Nurse

percent should be unsaturated fat, the fat that comes from vegetable sources, not the dangerous saturated fats (fats that are solid at room temperature and come from meat, whole milk products, and some oils).[5]

What's the problem with fat, you might ask? It has a nasty habit of killing us. We are not discussing obesity here. That's a separate problem. Even the thinnest person among us who eats a diet high in fats puts herself at risk.

Dietary fat is metabolized and transformed into that wonderful stuff called cholesterol. Cholesterol is nothing more or less than fat circulating in the blood. High enough concentrations of fat in the blood will invariably begin to leave deposits against the walls of the arteries. These deposits are called "plaque." When fat plaques build up in the coronary arteries, the arteries in the heart, they are the precursors of a heart attack. The heart attack and the subsequent heart disease are the Number One takers of life in the United States.

Further, fat plaques form in the carotid arteries, those big, throbbing arteries you can feel in your neck. They carry all the blood to the brain. If the tiniest fragment of that fat plaque should break off and be transported by the blood into your brain, where it then shuts off the flow of blood to

---

5   The Internet provides excellent information on nutrition and fat intake. See, for example, http://www.health.gov/dietaryguidelines/dga2005/recommendations.htm

The Five Rules for Long-Term Health

a part of the brain, you have had a stroke, the Number Two taker of life in the United States.

And if enough fat passes through your system for long enough, it can contribute to colon cancer, which is rapidly becoming the Number One cancer in the United States.

Finally, combine a high-fat diet and processed foods with lack of exercise, and you're dealing with the national crisis called obesity. The people of the United States are far and away the most obese population that has ever existed on planet Earth. It is this kind of obesity that is the foundation for Type 2, adult-onset diabetes.

Unless we choose differently, more than 70 percent of the people we work with, our families, and the people in our communities will die of one of four things: heart disease, stroke, cancer, and/or diabetes. We rarely any longer die of measles and mumps and chickenpox and diphtheria and polio and tuberculosis and scarlet fever and hundreds of other diseases. We no longer die from infected cuts or even from massive trauma. Medicine has gotten really good, and all that's left to take the lives of more than 70 percent of us are heart disease, stroke, cancer, and diabetes. And they are all related, at least in good part, to the massively high-fat American diet.

Consider that in 1970, Americans consumed an average

of 195 pounds of red meat and poultry per person. By 2007, though, that figure had gone to 221 pounds of red meat and poultry per person per year. No nation in history has consumed more meat than the United States. We must begin to limit that intake.

In my presentations, when I ask members of the audience, "Why do you love fat so much?" I get the answer "Because it tastes good."

"Yes, but why does it taste good?" Generally there is are only puzzled expressions around the room.

In order to understand why fat tastes good, please think of the bears up in the north woods. Each spring the bears comes out of their winter's hibernation. From that day until the day some months later when the bears return to hibernation, every bear, male or female, is thinking of only two things: sex and food. Now, the bear is not consciously thinking, "Boy, if I don't eat a lot and get fat before next winter comes, I'll probably starve to death in my den." No, this is not a matter of conscious thought at all. The bear, as we say, has an instinct. What does that mean? The bear is genetically programmed to certain eating behaviors.

Similarly, the birds sitting on the phone lines as autumn approaches are not thinking to themselves, "Boy, the days are getting short and they're getting cold. I'd better take off and

The Five Rules for Long-Term Health

fly south where it's warmer." No, the birds are genetically programmed to a specific behavior that is triggered by seasonal changes in their environment.

This is all very interesting, but what does it mean for us humans? The fact is that we are, like the bears, genetically programmed to get fat. Through all of human history, the primary taker of the lives of people—indeed, of whole populations—has been famine and starvation. In times of famine, those who are fat clearly have the highest chance for survival. We need fat. We crave fat. Therefore it tastes good.

Unlike any prior generations in human history, we are surrounded by an abundance of high-fat foods. Most of these foods are manufactured because the companies that make them know that we crave fat and will pay for fat. Our grandparents and great grandparents living on the farms and in the cities of the United States did not have the luxury of high-fat foods. It takes a tremendous amount of energy to create fat; before the advent of highly mechanized agriculture and industry, which has the capability to raise meat highly "marbled" with intramuscular fat, fat was a luxury.

In addition, government programs begun in the 1970s have provided massive subsidies to the farmers of the grains needed to grow cattle and pigs and chickens, the primary sources of our mounting meat consumption. Sadly, there has been not comparable subsidization of those who grow fruits and vegetables. Thus, I can go to the hospital cafeteria where I work and have a cheeseburger, French fries, ice cream, and soft drink for about $3.00. If, however, I go to the salad bar and make a really nice salad with lettuce, peas, mushrooms, and a few croutons, I can spend up to $4.50.[6]

My Dad Loved His Fat

When I was a boy, when we went out to dinner as a family, my dad would always order a T-bone steak. Restaurants in those days often bragged that their steaks actually hung over the edges of the plate. They did this primarily because the fat was not trimmed off the steaks. The steak came to the table completely surrounded with one-half to one inch of yellow fat. Dad would carefully, almost surgically, trim the fat from around his steak. The fat he pushed into a pile to the side. He would eat his steak, and then came the time to eat the fat. And if we kids didn't want all of our fat, he ate that, too.

At this point in my talks, I often notice members of the audience groaning and making faces of disgust at this picture. Please keep in mind that we now spend the most money for the highest quality steaks, which are high quality precisely because they are marbled. We have built the fat right into the meat and we love it. It's just that the people who sell us our meat don't refer to it as "intramuscular fat."

---

6   A book that I highly recommend is *The Omnivore's Dilemma* by Michael Pollan.

The Five Rules for Long-Term Health

The challenge to cutting the fat in the diet to no more than 25 percent of largely unsaturated fats is a genuine one. It will not be easy, because we are fundamentally addicted to fat. When I look at a restaurant menu and see on the left side a listing of all of the steaks and chops that are available and then see on the right side the listings of seafood, I have to almost force myself to stay focused on the right side of the menu because my instincts draw me almost irresistibly back over to those rich and delicious steaks and chops.

To illustrate how the manufacturers of food understand our addiction to fat, consider that you're driving down the highway. There on the side of the road is a billboard soaring high into the sky. The billboard is advertising a chain of restaurants. Does that the billboard portray a beautiful lettuce-and-cucumber salad with vinegar and oil dressing on the side? No, the billboard shows you the magnificent, double- or triple-thick beef burger with strips of bacon carefully laced across the top and cheese and special sauce running down the sides. A giant serving of French fries accompanies the burger.

Or perhaps the billboard shows you a huge slice of pizza with bubbly cheese and sausage and pepperoni covering the top. Possibly it shows you a thick beef burrito with juicy beef and sauce coming out of both ends. Dear reader, are you not salivating? We are so addicted to fat than just thinking about high-fat foods generates an arousal in us, and that arousal is shown by the fact that we salivate—salivation is our body's anticipation of eating.

Rule #3: If You Smoke, You Die

We can deal with this rule quickly. If you smoke, you die. Every smoker, with the possible exception of kids who think they are cool, knows that they are destroying their health. How could they not know it? These days smoking has become terribly expensive as well as the subject of increasing negative social pressure. As a result, almost everybody who smokes knows they should quit, and most are trying to quit.

How do I know this? I know this because there is a multibillion dollar industry that has grown up to sell smokers things to help them quit: patches and gums and hypnosis and support groups and so on. The only problem is that these things simply don't work unless a vital precondition has been met. The smoker who wants to quit really has to want to. The problem is that smokers generally want to quit the American Way: fast, easy, and cheap. So they go to the doctor and say, "Doctor, I want to quit smoking. Gimme some of them patches. My employer will pay for them."

But it doesn't work that way. A smoker who tries every known smoking cessation device that we have has a six-month quit rate of 19 percent. And that's pathetic. There is just one way to quit smoking and that is to quit. Oh, I grant that patches and gums and all the other stuff may help a smoker get through the first few hours or first couple of days. But we know full well that a smoker can put $5,000 worth of patches over every inch of flesh on his body and he will keep on smoking. Yet if he really wants to quit, he will do it. Some 50 million Americans have quit, and most did it before and without the aid of the devices that fundamentally don't work. They did it by quitting.

A Personal Comment

I took up smoking when I was 16 years old. My mom and dad smoked as well as most their friends. Our minister smoked. Our family doctor smoked. Radio (this was before television) programs were sponsored by cigarette companies. Everywhere you went, people were smoking: on the bus, in restaurants, and even in funeral homes. When I arrived at my college in 1952, there were upper-class students who had been hired by cigarette companies to hand out free samples of cigarettes to all the entering freshmen.

I'm not the kind of person to do things half way. From the time I started smoking, I smoked two or more packs of cigarettes each day. One brand of cigarettes gave you coupons with each pack. When you acquired enough coupons, you

That Guy Nurse

could trade them in for a radio or a tennis racket or hundreds of other items. When I became a professor, I started to smoke a pipe. It was very sophisticated.

As the years went by, I took up jogging, as did many others. Waking up in the morning, I would have a cup of coffee and a cigarette. I would leave the house and run five to seven miles. I would come home and have another cigarette and more coffee.

Finally, on a Saturday when I was 38 years old and as it was becoming quite clear that smoking was more than hazardous to your health—it could kill you—I decided to quit. I tore up my supply of cigarettes and threw out my pipe tobacco. I was one of the lucky ones. Never for a moment did I feel a desire to begin smoking again.

Then, years later, in my early 60s, I was on a long bike ride with a good friend. As we climbed a steep hill, he became quite alarmed. I was panting and gasping. He asked me what was wrong. I responded that nothing was wrong. I always had to breathe hard while climbing hills. Clearly agitated, he insisted that I see a doctor and have my lungs checked. So I did.

The results of the test to determine the health of my lungs revealed that I had emphysema. All my years of smoking had destroyed so much lung tissue that now that my lungs were more than 60 years old and developing a sort of stiffness that can come with age—they were no longer capable of passing enough oxygen into my blood. Exertion left me winded. My heart had to work harder to pump enough blood to pick up enough oxygen to keep me going. Now, as much as I love my biking and my kayaking, my activities are increasingly restricted. My condition is not going to improve.

I would like to blame the cigarette companies and the advertising agencies for my problem. The simple fact, however, is that I did this to myself.

My problem with smokers is not that they're going to die. They cannot help but know that this is the long-term outcome of smoking. My problem is not that the smoker is going to bring terrible pain and suffering and maybe bankruptcy to his family. Again, how could the smoker not know that this is another one of the outcomes of smoking. No, that's a choice the smoker makes. No, what bugs me about smoking is this: it will cost between $170,000 and $350,000 for the smoker to die. That's how much medical care is going to be invested, on average, before the smoker dies, plus all of the costs of lost productivity to America's businesses.

If the smoking causes lung cancer, its most common outcome, the smoker does not die right away. No, the smoker comes into the hospital where surgeons open the chest and remove the portion of lung that has a tumor. Then the chest is closed and the smoker receives chemo or radiation therapy. And when the cancer returns, as it almost always does and certainly if the smoker does not quit smoking, the chest will be opened the second time and more lung removed. This can be done two or three times before there is not enough lung left to live on or the cancer metastasizes.

If the smoking should cause heart disease, I've already described the things we do to control heart disease. As a cardiac nurse, I have cared for patients having their third open-heart surgery because they smoked. That's up to a quarter of a million dollars right there.

What bugs me is that the smoker doesn't have to pay it. If the smoker is employed, the employer pays. That means that all the other employees in the company pay in reduced wages and benefits. It also means that the customers of the company pay the increased prices charged for the company's products. If the employee should survive the company and go on Medicare, then we all chip in as taxpayers to pay for their care. And that's simply not fair.

Rule #4: Drink Alcohol (in Moderation)

This is the rule that most people like. There has to be some good news somewhere in this whole thing! Rule #4 says that if you genuinely care about your health, you will probably have a drink tonight. Because, you see, a drink each day can have some very nice health benefits. They're not great health benefits, but then again, most of us don't need a big excuse.

What am I talking about here? A drink every day is going to help both the good and the bad cholesterols improve. A drink every day slows down the aging process so you live a little bit longer. A drink every day helps take some of the stress out of life. If you don't deal with stress, and we all do have stress, it can eventually tear down the immune system and make us vulnerable to some very bad things. The only truly effective way to deal with stress is, of course, exercise. But from a medical point of view, it might be a good idea after exercise to enjoy a drink.

Now, how much am I talking about? Well, a glass and a half or two glasses of wine is just about perfect. In Wisconsin, a couple of bottles of beer isn't too shabby. It's a little calorific, though. Years ago my own doctor ordered me to have a martini each day. I care deeply about my health, and so each night, generally just before supper, I force myself to have a martini.

Here are the rules. (There are always rules, aren't there?) If you are alcoholic or in any way allergic to alcohol, you cannot drink—it will kill you. If you believe, for whatever reason, that drinking is wrong, don't do it. It will just add stress to your life. If you're going to operate any kind of a vehicle or show up at work, you cannot drink because that would be flat-out stupid. Are we clear?

Rule #5: Do Preventive Maintenance

That brings us to Rule #5. It may be the last but it is far from least important. Each and every one of us has something available to us that our parents and grandparents never had. We can, if we choose, have our own customized personal schedule for preventive maintenance.

"Preventive maintenance": we all understand it and we all practice it. If you own an automobile, you do preventive maintenance. You look at the schedule that comes with your car that tells you that every 3000 or 5000 or 10,000 miles you need to change the oil or rotate the tires or change the transmission fluid or give the engine a tune-up. And you know that if you follow the rules of preventive maintenance, with a little luck and unless you do something really stupid, your car or whatever other piece of machinery you may be dealing with can last almost forever. Ignore preventive maintenance and you can reduce the best car or snowmobile or boat in the world into junk in just a few months.

Recently we did not have the medical knowledge or skills to practice a high-level of preventive health maintenance. But today we do have it. And as in the case of each of the things we have been discussing, we have to choose. If we choose to practice preventive health maintenance, our first step is to research as much as we can of our family medical histories. Why family medical history? Think of it this way:

An Apple a Day . . .

Now complete the following sentence: "An apple a day..."[7] That's what we learned from our parents and what they learned from their parents: take care of yourself, eat an apple every day, and with any luck, you may be able to go

---

The Alligators in Your Swamp

You are walking through a swamp. It's midnight. It's foggy. And you don't know where the alligators are. That's not a good situation. I don't into the swamp unless I know what are the alligators are. Do you have the cholesterol alligator? The high blood pressure alligator? The diabetes alligator? The heart disease alligator? The depression alligator? The cancer alligator? There are lots of alligators living in your swamp, and your family medical history provides you with insight into the ones you'll have to have to deal with. So you begin by researching your family medical history of at least mom and dad, brothers and sisters, and aunts and uncles and cousins as well as your own. Any history you can gather beyond this is frosting on the cake and well worth having.

---

7   "keeps the doctor away."

from the cradle to the grave, from the womb to the tomb, and never have to see a doctor, because the only reason to see a doctor is that something is broken, burning, bleeding, oozing, or in pain.

And guess what? For our parents, that was exactly how to think about doctors and medicine. Take care of yourself and you may never have to take medicine or see a doctor. But that world is gone, long gone. Today we all need to have a doctor not as a mechanic to fix things but as a coach and mentor in ensuring our long-term health.

So you do your family medical history, as much as you can, and you go to your doctor and say, "Doctor, I would like my preventive maintenance plan. Tell me, based on my age, my gender, and my history, how often I should come to see you to receive diagnostic checks and tests and to receive the information that will allow me to stay healthy and to find any threats and fix them before they get to the point where they can kill me." I'll be saying a lot more about this in Section II of this book, "The Professional Patient."

I do not want to underestimate the difficulty with the practice of prevention and early detection. There's an old saying, "Denial ain't just a river in Egypt." Given the difficulty of seeing the doctor, the expense of seeing the doctor, and the very normal fear that the doctor may find something bad,

Americans by the tens of millions do not actively practice early detection and intervention. They ignore symptoms until the symptoms become so bad they have no choice but to be seen by a doctor. And that's when the message is too often, "I'm sorry, the cancer is metastasized" or "You had a massive heart attack and there's nothing we can do." **It takes courage and commitment to practice preventive health care.**

Probably the greatest and least appreciated development in modern medical knowledge and skill is that we can prevent most of the things that can take our lives before the end of our lifespan. And what we cannot prevent, we can detect early enough to fix. But as with each and every thing we've talked about so far in this book, you have to make the choice.

So there it is: you're going to live a long time. You won't be allowed to die. But if you choose to engage in regular exercise, limit the amount of fat in your diet, don't even think about smoking, enjoy a drink responsibly and in moderation, and form a partnership with your doctor to practice prevention and early detection, then, after 90 to 95 years or maybe even a little more, you will die. But the odds get awfully, awfully good that you will die healthy.

That is exactly the way it's supposed to be.

notes:

_____

_____

_____

_____

_____

_____

_____

_____

_____

_____

_____

_____

_____

_____

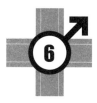

You Are the President and CEO of Your Own Life

If you remember anything from Part I of this book (and I hope you do!), it should be that you are going to live a very long time. All other things being equal, you will not be allowed to die. If, then, you choose to live your life in good health, you must, in addition to practicing a healthy lifestyle, become a **Professional Patient**.

You ask, what is a Professional P atient? What I mean by that term is that everyone in one way or another is a patient or will be a patient in the American medical system. You will be a patient seeking cure for sickness or repair of injury. You will be a patient seeking knowledge and/or preventive care. But you will be a patient, and there are better and worse ways to be a patient.

The better way is to think of yourself as the president of your life. You are the chief executive officer, the CEO of your life. You may choose to delegate your authority to somebody else, but in that case, you have turned your life over to another person. That, generally, is not a good idea. The president of the United States appoints a group of Cabinet officers. They have no executive authority by themselves. They serve as advisers to the president. As long as their advice is good and useful, the president normally retains their services. When, however, they prove to be no longer useful, they are replaced. They serve, as it is said, "at the pleasure of the president."

Thought of in this way you, as president of your own life, also have a cabinet. You may have an attorney, your secretary of law. If you have a doctor, that is your secretary of health. Your real estate broker, the person you hire to remodel your kitchen, the landscaper, your personal fitness trainer, and everyone else you employ, permanently or temporarily, full time or part time, they are all your cabinet and you are the CEO. Just like the Cabinet members in Washington, your cabinet exists to advise you and to serve you. But you are always the president, the person in charge.

President Harry S Truman had a sign on his desk in the Oval Office, "The Buck Stops Here." What was true for Truman is true for you. In matters of your health, you are ultimately responsible. When you have your health, you are responsible for maintaining and improving it. And when, for whatever reason, you become sick or injured, you and only you are responsible for the decisions that are intended to restore you to health. Your doctor is your advisor. You may choose to accept his advice or you may seek a second opinion or third opinion. But whatever you do, the final choice belongs to you and you alone. Recognizing that situations such as serious illness or injury can happen, you may (should) designate someone to hold your Durable Power of Attorney for Health Care.[1] The decision to do this and the person you choose are also the actions of a CEO.

So you need to be professional about this. Let's examine what it means to be a professional. I am using the term "professional" to refer to a person who has brought together a body of knowledge and skills and merged them in such a way as to be able to accomplish a task or to achieve a goal. In Green Bay, we have a football team, the Green Bay Packers (Go, Pack!). They are professionals. Each player has a body of knowledge and skills that are used to accomplish the goals of the team. If any one of us were to walk onto the practice field and attempt to take the place of one of those players, we would, unquestionably, fail. In fact we would be lucky to survive. We lack the knowledge and skills that make them

---

1   See Chaper 13 for informaiton about the Durable Power of Attorney for Health Care.

You Are the President and CEO of Your Own Life

professionals in their field.

Each of you reading this book is a professional at something. You possess the knowledge and skills that allow you to do something. If I were to attempt to do any one of your professional tasks, I would, in all likelihood, fail. I lack the knowledge and skills that you have to do what you do. If, on the other hand, you were to come to my hospital and attempt to transfuse a pint of blood, dress a surgical incision, or start an IV line, you would, in all likelihood, also fail.

So when it comes to matters of our own health, we must all become professionals; we must acquire the knowledge and skills necessary in order to use the American medical system to our advantage—and, unfortunately, too often to protect ourselves from it. This section of the book discusses how you can—and why you should—become a Professional Patient.

Know Your Family Medical History

The first kind of knowledge that a Professional Patient has relates to family medical history. Why is family medical history an important piece of knowledge? As I explained in Chapter 5, if we don't know our family medical history, it's like walking through a swamp on a dark, foggy night with no moon and you will have don't know where the alligators

A Family with A History

Just a few months ago, I was shocked to read in the paper that the 41-year-old son of some very dear friends had been found dead in his bed. He was an active outdoorsman and worked in a construction job. Rosalie and I went to the visitation at the funeral home. I went to his father and gave him a hug. He said, "We have good news." I thought, "What could possibly be good about this?" He then said, "He died of a heart attack. But he never saw a doctor." Then I understood. A 41-year-old man with an active lifestyle is found dead in bed. Drugs? Violence? Suicide? What? A heart attack is something we can understand.

Now, here's the problem. Dad has had two open heart surgeries and currently has a pacemaker in his chest to keep his heart in rhythm. Mom has also had open heart surgery. But nobody thought to insist that all of their kids see a cardiologist. This young man had five serious coronary artery blockages. They did not develop in a matter of weeks or months or even a few years. They took a long, long time to become lethal and could have been detected and corrected at any point along the way.

I can understand that Mom and Dad may not have recognized the importance of family history. I cannot understand or accept that neither the family doctor nor the cardiologists and surgeons they saw along the way informed them and encouraged them to make sure their children were directed to somebody who could have detected the danger and fixed it. Unfortunately, the parents were amateurs—not Professional Patients—and their son is dead.

are. Knowing your family medical history tells you about the alligators that live in your swamp—the cholesterol alligator, the high blood pressure alligator, the diabetes alligator, the heart disease alligator, the depression alligator, the cancer alligator, etc. Armed with this information, you can begin to exploit the capacity of the American medical system not just to cure or repair you when necessary but, more importantly, to help you stay healthy.

Having a family history of, let's say, cancer does not mean that you will one day have cancer. Having a family history of heart disease does not mean that you will one day have heart disease. **Family history shows us tendency, not destiny.**

A final note about medical records is in order here. Most of us have, over our lifetimes, seen many doctors in many places. We have medical records spread over the country in lots of clinics and hospitals. It may surprise you to know that those records all belong to you. That's the law. If you have a significant medical history, especially if you have one or more chronic conditions, you should keep a copy of those records with you. The various clinics and hospitals where your records are being kept are entitled to charge a reasonable fee for duplicating those records and getting them to you. Yet for your own protection and as a partner with whatever doctor(s) you are now are seeing or will see in the future, you should gather all of your records and make them available to your doctor(s).

Find a Physician Partner

Also in Chapter 5, I asked you to complete the following sentence: "An apple a day . . . " to make the point that we were taught by our parents that if we took care of ourselves, we may never have to see a doctor. They lived at a time and with a medical system in which this sentiment was precisely the right way to think—that is, if you take care of yourself by, for example, eating an apple every day, then with a little luck and unless you so something really stupid, you might be able to go through your entire life without ever having to see a doctor.

After all, in prior generations, one only went to see the doctor if one was sick or injured. And, as I have said, then there was very little the doctor could do. The prevalence of this belief about staying away from doctors is made clear to me time and time again as I am told, usually by men—and men who take great pride in the utterance—"Well, I haven't seen a doctor in 10 years." What they're saying is that they have not been sick or injured in 10 years and, given that fact, there was no need whatsoever to have to see a doctor. President George W. Bush gave evidence of his belief in the "Apple a Day" dictum when he stated that America does have universal health coverage because anybody can go to

You Are the President and CEO of Your Own Life

the emergency room.[2]

Only within the past few decades has medical knowledge allowed us to understand how to prevent conditions that were, for prior generations, almost always fatal. Only within the past few decades have medical knowledge and technology advanced to the point where we can detect heretofore dangerous conditions early enough to prevent them from becoming lethal. This is the heart of the concept of prevention. There is a solid evidence that up to 70 percent of all medical expense is related to the treatment of conditions that are, in principle, preventable. This includes, of course, problems related to obesity, smoking, excessive use of alcohol, and failure to exercise. Adopting a healthy lifestyle will substantially improve the odds of staying healthy for a long time.

At the same time, though, the Professional Patient uses the power of medicine to provide for the early detection of medical conditions that could eventually be fatal if not detected early enough. Early detection, then, is the second major component of long-term health after knowing family medical history. The Professional Patient understands this and is prepared to exploit this capacity.

---

2   On July 22, 2007, President Bush stated, "People have access to health care in America. After all, just go to the Emergency Room." President Bush, like many Americans, believed that the purpose of the health care system is to cure and to repair, not to promote health or preventive care.

The first step is to form a partnership with a physician, a partnership designed to provide preventive care and information on health rather than only to provide treatment for sickness and injury. You'll learn more about this in the chapter on the doctor/patient relationship, Chapter 9.

Fluffy

Student nurses are required to have an understanding of anatomy and physiology. Anatomy is the study of the body's structure. Physiology is the study of how the body's systems work. As nursing students, we did not have an actual human body to study, a cadaver. Rather, we were given a cat's cadaver. In teams of four, we studied our cat and slowly and systematically dissected its body to learn about bones and muscle and all the body's organs. Our cat's name was Fluffy.

In the oftentimes callous way of students who were more than a little afraid of and in wonder of the body that they were dissecting and studying, we gave Fluffy a personality and a life history. Fluffy had been a barn cat but was always very gentle with children and was appreciated as a great mouser around the farm. Unfortunately, one day Fluffy wandered off and was picked up by the animal control people, taken to a shelter, and then, when nobody came to get her, was euthanized.

135

You Are the President and CEO of Your Own Life

As we slowly cut Fluffy apart, making notes about and discussing each new discovery, we came to appreciate many things. We came to appreciate the almost unbelievable complexity and beauty of what was once a living creature. For me, I found an entirely new appreciation for the skill of the surgeon. It took a deftness of touch far beyond my meager abilities to separate the various muscle tissues of Fluffy's body without mangling them. The textbook would show me pictures of what I was looking for, but even after I had done my most skillful work, it was almost impossible to find what the textbook assured me was right in front of my face.

I will never forget Fluffy. Often, as I am caring for a patient—dressing an incision, doing range of motion therapy on arms or legs, giving an injection, starting an IV, or drawing blood—I cannot help but think about and admire what I now understand to be the magnificent complexity that lies just under my hands as well as the almost unbelievable skill of the surgeons who can remove, repair, and replace the parts of this complex organism.

Before I leave Fluffy, I want to tell you about a wonderful opportunity to discover the magnificent beauty and complexity of the human body. There is an exhibition called "Body Worlds" (www.bodyworlds.com), which puts on display wonderfully preserved human bodies. Various bodies are shown in ways that demonstrate muscles and joints, the internal organs, the brain, and the bones as well as the nervous system. Although this exhibition has generated controversy where ever it goes, I believe that it is truly one of the most informative and remarkable experiences one can have. The power of this exhibition is demonstrated to me each time I attend. There are always dozens and even hundreds of high school students attending on field trips. Past experience tells me that high school students on field trips are generally noisy and engaged in horseplay. Yet at every Body Worlds exhibition I have attended, the students demonstrate an almost unbelievable attentive quiet and even reverence toward what they are seeing. If you ever have an opportunity to attend a Body Worlds exhibition, I highly recommend that you do.

Know How Your Body Works

The Professional Patient also has a basic understanding of the human body and how it works. I am convinced that the great majority of people know far more about how their cars work than they do about their own bodies.

People almost always become experts about a disease or the consequences of an injury after they have the disease or have suffered the injury. That's the time they go running to the library or online in an effort to understand what has happened and what may happen. This is understandable, because most of us tend to take the condition of being healthy for granted. We give lip service to the saying, "If you haven't got your health, you haven't got anything," and then we engage in the very behaviors that are likely to destroy our health. The Professional Patient, though, armed first with an understanding of family history, and then in partnership with a doctor, comes to understand bad things before they happen and uses this understanding to prevent them. Unfortunately, most of us are amateurs, even illiterate, when it comes to understanding our bodies and how to keep them healthy.

In my presentations, I illustrate this point in this way, after selecting someone from the audience:

Me: Tell me, have you ever cut your finger?

Audience Member: Yes, I have.

Me: Well, what happens?

A.M.: It bleeds.

Me: Now, if you just stand and watch it bleed, does all the blood drain out of your body until you die?

A.M.: No. It stops.

Me: What makes it stop?   At this point and the answer is either, "I don't know" or "It clots."

That Guy Nurse

Me: What makes it clot?

A.M.: I don't know.

All of this dialogue leads into a discussion of how blood clots. When you cut your finger, the red stuff that comes oozing out isn't just red stuff. It has lots of different components. Your blood contains white cells, whose job is to fight off infection. Blood also contains cells whose job it is to pick up molecules of oxygen in your lungs and deliver them to cells throughout your body. Without a supply of that oxygen, the cells that compose our bodies could not survive. Circulating blood is what keeps you alive.

There is a third group of cells, called platelets. Their job is to keep you from bleeding to death. When you get a cut on your finger or anywhere else on your body, even on the inside, your body's systems mobilize groups of platelets and send them to the point where there is a lesion, a break. Once there, they are like the little Dutch boy with his finger in the dike. They block up the cut or lesion. When they are exposed to air, they dry and form a hard crust. We call that a scab. Underneath, then, another process gets underway to repair or replace the cells that were damaged. So we don't bleed to death unless, of course, we are hemophiliacs whose blood lacks the ability to clot.

You Are the President and CEO of Your Own Life

"Well," you say, "that's all very interesting but so what? What makes it important information for me?"

Most people, including myself before I went to nursing school, thought that heart attacks occurred when a coronary artery got blocked. I thought that there would be a slow buildup of fat plaques in the artery until one day the last molecule of fat fell into place and blocked the artery and caused a heart attack. But that's not the way it works. More than 80 percent of all heart attacks occur in people who do not have a coronary blockage greater than 30 percent.

"Well, then," you ask, "what causes a heart attack?"

The answer is that the person with a heart attack had a plaque deposit on the wall of a coronary artery that became inflamed and ruptured. Our bodies treat that situation exactly like the cut on the finger. They rush platelets to the scene to heal the lesion in the wall of the artery. The platelets, being big and sticky, get to the scene and form a clot, and the clot blocks the artery and there is a heart attack.

Now, having been given this information, I ask my audiences, "How many of you take a baby aspirin every day?" Normally five to 10 percent of the audience raise their hands.

You might want to know that taking a little 81 mg baby

aspirin every day can reduce your risk of a heart attack, the Number One taker of life in the United States, by better than 70 percent. The aspirin does two things. First, it has an anti-coagulant property. It reduces the likelihood that if you do have a lesion in a coronary artery, the subsequent blood clot will be large enough to block the artery. Second, and more important, aspirin is an anti-inflammatory. It reduces the risk that you will have the kind of inflammation that can rupture a coronary plaque.

Now, I am not telling you to take a baby aspirin every day. I am not your physician. I don't know your medical history. I don't know what other medications you may be taking right now. I will say that the Professional Patient, having been given a piece of information like this, probably calls his or her doctor and asks, "Should I be taking a baby aspirin every day?" The odds are very good your doctor will say something like, "You mean you aren't?" Often times physicians think that we know more than we do, that we are more professional than we are. Most often the people who raised their hands tell me that their doctor told them to take a baby aspirin, but when I ask if the doctor explained why, the answer is usually "no."

Back to the idea that the Professional Patient understands the body and how it works. This does not need to be the kind of understanding that a physician or other trained

141

health professional has. But it has to be an understanding of at least the basics of anatomy and physiology. Without such an understanding, it is hard if not impossible to know what is required to keep the body functioning well and, perhaps more important, to recognize when things have gone wrong. Lack of such an understanding complicates your attempt to explain to the doctor what is wrong as well as complicating the ability to understand and appreciate the doctor's diagnosis and recommended plan of treatment.

Here's another example, probably even more relevant for those of us who live relatively sedentary lives. I'll start with a question: How does the blood in a person's big toe get back to the heart where it can pick up more oxygen and be recirculated? Almost everybody believes (as did I until I went to nursing school) that the heart pumps the blood throughout the body—very much like the pump in a swimming pool. Water is pumped out of the pool and through a filter and back into the pool again. But it's not quite that way in the human circulatory system.

When the heart contracts, it forces blood into and through the lungs and then out into the rest of the body. It's easy to feel the pumping action of the heart by pressing your fingers against your wrist or on either side of the neck. The force of blood rushing through the arteries close to the heart is called a pulse. However, by the time blood has reached the furthest extremities of the body, the initial pressure provided by the pumping heart has been dissipated. There is not enough pressure left to move the blood from the foot up through the leg to the torso and back to the heart. The actual mechanism by which blood is returned is far more complex and far more interesting.

When the a blood cell reaches its final destination, say in the big toe, there is just enough residual pressure left to move the cell through the walls of a nearby vein. The human body contains (can you believe this?) more than 60,000 miles of veins, arteries, and capillaries. Those vessels are contained in our muscle tissue. All of the body's muscles are perfused (contain all those thousands of miles) with veins.

In the lower half of the body, the veins themselves contain thousands of tiny, one-way valves. These valves operate much in the manner of a tube of toothpaste. If you squeeze a tube of toothpaste with the cap on, nothing happens. Take the cap off and squeeze it and you get toothpaste. If you cut the bottom off the tube and squeeze, then toothpaste comes out of both ends. The valves in the veins act just like the cap on the toothpaste tube. They allow the blood to flow in only one direction—toward the heart. We move our bodies by contracting muscles. Walking, coughing, stretching, and any other bodily motion is achieved through the contraction of muscles. When muscles contract, they squeeze the veins in the muscle tissue. The blood can flow in only one direction—toward the heart. And that is how the circulatory system works.

Why is this important? Well, unless we are moving, the blood does not move. And blood that doesn't move has the nasty habit of forming clots. And clots have the nasty habit of causing death through stroke or pulmonary embolism (a blood clot in the lungs). For a great many Americans today, daily life does not involve much moving. We sit, sometimes for hours, at computer terminals or at desks. We sit, sometimes for hours, in front of the television. In factories, machine operators can sit, sometimes for an entire shift, just monitoring the machines. We sit in movie theaters and on long plane flights.

The Professional Patient understands the importance of moving. The Professional Patient makes sure to get up and move around a bit. On a long car ride, the Professional Patient does not drive five or six hours until the car needs gas (or until the driver or passenger needs a restroom stop, which at my age is pretty often!). The Professional Patient stops every hour or so, gets out, and takes a quick walk around the car. The Professional Patient working at a desk makes sure to get up and move at least every hour or so. In short, we have to move!

That Guy Nurse

There are many easy and interesting ways to learn about the body and how it works. The Web site www.WebMD.com, for example, is an excellent source of information. The National Institutes of Health (Google "NIH") is another great place to go. One caution about going to the Internet for medical information, though, is to be aware of the source of that information. Many health-related Web sites are little more than advertisements. The Professional Patient "vets" any source of information.

Finally, as I said at the beginning of this chapter, it seems to me that people go to the Web or to the library to get information about some health issue only after their health has been compromised. The heart attack has occurred. The cancer is been detected. Then the rush is on to learn all there is to know about that condition. Given, though, what we know about the prevention of health risks—especially those in our own families—this is more than a little like locking the barn after the horse has been stolen.

Recognize and Describe Symptoms

The Professional Patient is able to recognize the symptoms that something is not working the way it should, and the Professional Patient, recognizing a symptom, pays attention to it. The Professional Patient may even keep a diary of the history of a symptom or symptoms.

Here is a common scenario played out in the lives of doctors and nurses. The patient, call him Tom, arrives at the clinic. The first task facing the doctor is to find out why Tom has sought an appointment.

"Tom, why have you come in today?"

"Doc, I'm in a lot of pain."

"Tell me, Tom, on a scale of one to 10, 10 being the worst pain you can imagine, how bad is your pain?"

Tom is clearly thinking the question over and he responds, "14."

When I first started my nursing career, I would get very frustrated at what I took to be a smart-ass answer to a very straightforward question. Then I realized that Tom and most other patients did not know why the doctor was asking the question. Tom thought to himself, "Well, he wants to know what kind of pain I'm in. I could tell him '6' but what does that mean? That could be his '2' or his '9.' I want him to know that I'm really in pain so I'm going to tell him '14.'"

What nobody explained to Tom is that this question is the first of a series of questions designed to identify the cause of the pain. Pain is, of course, a symptom. There are lots of ways of relieving or eliminating pain. In fact, many amateurs, experiencing pain, immediately rush to the drugstore to buy any one of a variety of products designed to relieve pain. But that's the amateur. The Professional Patient realizes that the pain is a part of the body saying, "Hey, over here damn it, pay attention to me."

The first task of the doctor is to determine what's causing the pain, and the question about the severity of the pain provides baseline information. Once the doctor thinks she has found the cause of the pain, she begins to treat it. If, after treatment begins and the patient who first reported the pain to be a 6 reports that it's now a 9, that's a pretty good indication that the cause is still a mystery. If, on the other hand, the patient says that the pain is gone, that's a good indication that the doctor figured it out. Either way the question is a serious one, and a Professional Patient gives it a serious answer.

The question about the severity of the pain is followed by other questions. "Where is the pain located?" In response, often Tom will merely indicate some general area of his body. This is of very little use to the doctor. When asked how long he has had the pain, Tom replies, "a long time." But what is "a long time?" Two hours? Two days? Two months?

Tom may be asked what kind of pain it is, and often he doesn't have the vaguest idea of what the question is about The doctor is asking if it's a burning pain, a stabbing pain, a

You Are the President and CEO of Your Own Life

throbbing pain, a constant pain, or an intermittent pain. The kind of pain can be an important clue as to the cause of the pain, and the Professional Patient gives careful thought to identifying the character of the pain.

A professional answer to the question about pain may go something like this:

"I made this appointment because I have a lot of pain. Right now I'd rate my pain as a 6. It's over here on my right side, just below my ribs. It's not on the outside. I can poke myself over here and it doesn't hurt. The hurt seems to be way inside. It's a stabbing pain. It's like somebody put a knife in there.

"And it's constant, it's always there. I first noticed it last Tuesday. When I woke up, I was aware that something didn't feel quite right over there on my right side just below my ribs. It really wasn't even a pain. It just didn't feel right. I ignored it, but then on Thursday morning when I woke up, it was the same sensation, only now it hurt. I guess it was about a 2. I thought I should probably see you about it, but by the time I got my teeth brushed, it was gone. Then, this morning it woke me up. A stabbing pain under the ribs on the right side and it was a least a 6. I called for an appointment, and when I got in the car to come in and bent over to my right to fasten my seatbelt, the pain disappeared. But as soon as I sat up straight again, it was back."

In just a few seconds, the Professional Patient has given his doctor volumes of information about his symptom, pain. Based on that information, the doctor is able to immediately eliminate hundreds of possible causes of pain. She can begin to focus attention on only the very few that would cause pain of increasing intensity over the period of a week in that particular location and having that specific character and intensity, including being relieved by a specific postural change. The doctor can now get focused on the few things that would cause the history that the patient has related.

Most everyone has known a certian kind of person. In my experience, and at the risk of not being politically correct, I would suggest this person is almost always a woman. At parties, she bores everyone to death with stories about the mysterious medical condition she has. She has seen five different doctors and none of them has been able to figure out what's wrong. She is so proud!

Now, it may be that she saw five stupid doctors. It may even be that she does have some rare condition that nobody can figure out. The greatest likelihood, however, is that each of the five doctors she saw received an ambiguous, partial, incomplete, and even erroneous description of her symptoms. As a result, each doctor had to guess. The last thing a Professional Patient wants is to have the doctor guessing.

How, When, and Where to Enter the Medical System

The amateur patient is likely to enter the medical system at the wrong time and at the wrong place. The result of this is that problems last longer and that far too often the end of treatment is marked by prolonged illness or disability and even death. The amateur patient fears the doctor, fears the cost of co-payments and deductibles, and fears receiving bad news. Doctors cause pain and embarrassment. They put their fingers where fingers do not belong. They ask questions that the amateur patient does not want to answer or that he must lie to answer. "How many packs a day do you smoke?" "One." It is a matter of habit and long experience, that the doctor may automatically write a 2 or a 3 in the patient's chart. "How much to you drink each day?" "Generally I have a beer or two or a cocktail." This will may recorded as "a six-pack per day" or "3-4 drinks a day."

Patients who enter the medical system too soon waste their money and the system's resources. Patients who enter the system too late endanger their health and their lives. Plus, the treatment of their problems becomes far more expensive, since the problems have become more serious and the treatments more time consuming and requiring greater resources.

Ask-A-Nurse

The Professional Patient begins with an adequate knowledge of the symptoms of various medical problems as well as the most appropriate response to those symptoms. Even with this knowledge, however, there will be situations in which the symptoms are confusing or in which it is unclear if and when to contact the medical system. In many communities and with many different insurance programs, it is possible to call a service like "ask-a-nurse." The nurses staffing these programs are provided with an extensive computerized database of symptoms and the most appropriate responses. They are trained to ask the right questions and then to give the most appropriate advice: "Rest and call your doctor in the morning," "Go to the nearest urgent care," "Hang up the phone and call 911 now!" One of the most unappreciated and underused and yet most valuable medical services we have is the ask-a-nurse program. The Professional Patient knows this and uses it.

You Are the President and CEO of Your Own Life

notes:

_____

_____

_____

_____

_____

_____

_____

_____

_____

_____

_____

_____

_____

_____

_____

That Guy Nurse

The American System:
Not About Health and Wellness

Over and over and over we hear talk about America's "health care" system. Yet as I said earlier, we do not have a health care system. What we have is a medical system. Further, it is a system whose components—insurance companies, hospital systems, pharmaceutical companies, and companies that design and build medical hardware, from scanners to prosthetics—have as a driving purpose to generate profit. Now, there is nothing wrong with profit. I tried to make a profit in my work as a professor, as an executive director, as a nurse, and as a speaker. I hope to make a profit from sales of this book. Yet too often the goal of profit is not consistent with the goal of good health. There is a conflict of interest that lies very close to the heart of the American medical system.

One of the primary purposes of this book is to make this point very clear. Why? Because health, that condition that is so fundamental to happiness, is, when all is said and done, the responsibility of each individual for himself or herself. The medical system can do things undreamed of only half a century ago to cure illness and repair trauma. But without the knowledgeable and active participation of its patients, it does and will continue to fail to be a system that promotes health.

The "Corporatization" of the American Medical System

One of the saddest consequences of the "corporatization" of the American medical system has been the demise of primary care. Beginning largely in the 1980s, the American medical system came not just to resemble but to operate as a corporate business—a business whose goal and whose driving force was profit. And, as I have stated earlier, there is no money in health. A medical system requires illness, both chronic and acute, and trauma in order to generate profit. Without these, there is little market for expensive medicines, expensive equipment, expensive hospitals, and expensive surgeries.

Primary care medicine, on the other hand, is fundamentally the medicine of health, of prevention, and of early detection. Before the advent of today's medical and pharmaceutical technologies, the primary care doctor did treat illness and try to repair trauma but with few resources. His goal was to keep his patients healthy. But even then there was little he could do. We had a few of the sophisticated tools available today to do early detection. We did not even have the knowledge we have today about the value of exercise. Our knowledge of nutrition was as limited as today's choices of foods, natural and processed, is expansive. Then, just as science gave us more knowledge about the causes of diseases and how to treat them, about the importance of exercise, and about the value of nutrition, and even, after a long struggle, knowledge of the fact that cigarettes kill, we failed. We failed to see that the new knowledge could be useful in teaching people how to maintain their health, useful in developing prevention as a core of medical practice, useful in exploiting the ability to detect problems early before they became serious.

Now, back to primary care. Primary care is the doorway into the medical system. Fifty years ago primary care was what medicine was all about. Today, though, primary care medicine has been relegated to being the gateway to the world of the specialists. For doctors in family practice, internal medicine, and pediatrics, income has been shrinking. These doctors are generally required to see 25 or more patients each day and thus are allowed to spend only a few minutes with each. Because of this, the role of the primary care physician as a teacher and as the provider of preventive medicine has been seriously degraded.

The American System:
Not About Health and Wellness

Consider median compensation for physicians in the United States in 2009: family practice, $197,655, cardiac surgery, $507,143, anesthesiology, $366.640, diagnostic radiology, $478.000, orthopedic surgery for joint replacement, $580,711, opthalmology, $326,384. Is it any wonder that few prospective doctors choose primary care?

Add to this that from a medical point of view, most people in the United States are functionally illiterate. The best evidence I can give for this sad fact is that Americans annually spend billions of dollars on medical products that make promises that could not conceivably be fulfilled and that lack any foundation in scientific inquiry whatsoever.[1] Further evidence is provided by the knowledge that up to 70 percent of all the money being spent on medical care is for the treatment of preventable conditions. Prevention and early detection should be the primary activities of a genuine "health care" system. Prevention and early detection would be the first things sought by a people who are medically literate.

As I said earlier, it was terrible to realize early in my nursing experience that most of my patients were their own victims.

---

1   Virtually all of the thousands of medical products advertised on television, on the Internet, and in newspapers and magazines claim that they are based on "scientific research." Sadly, a quick look at the National Institutes of Health will reveal that these claims are simply false. Often the "scientists" who are quoted and who did the research were in the employ of the very company whose product is being touted in the advertisement.

They were on the cardiac floor or in hospice because the decisions they had made and the lifestyles they had chosen brought them there. I don't know of anybody who wakes up in the morning and says to himself, "I think I'll go out today and engage in activities that will destroy my health." And yet that is exactly what we do by the tens of millions every day. If we are and must be the CEOs of our own lives, most of us are driving our companies into bankruptcy and ruin.

To a large degree, this sad situation is a product of the fact that what was once a close and extended relationship between doctor and patient has become a fundamentally commercial relationship between "consumers" and "providers." The "bean counters," the accountants and managers, have largely taken control of the American medical system. Doctors, especially primary care doctors, are told what medications they can prescribe, what procedures they can recommend, and, most importantly, how much time they can spend with each patient. And since most patients generally simply accept the doctor's recommendations, the system moves on.

It has been my experience that many primary care doctors find their situation to be more than frustrating. As one doctor said to me, "They taught me to practice medicine when I was in medical school, but when I came out into the world, I wasn't allowed to do it."

The American System:
Not About Health and Wellness

The result is an ironic (and scary) contradiction: at the same time that the knowledge we have of medicine and healing and health is increasing in quantum leaps, the time that the primary care doctor has to spend with patients is deceasing proportionately. The "specialists" are not in the business of—nor are they expected to be—spending time listening to or teaching their patients. Their job is to do what specialists do: treat medical conditions. As a result, we continue to be a nation wasting its health while paying ruinous amounts of money in efforts to restore it.

Welcome to the Era of "Hamster Medicine"

In my presentations, I illustrate the concept of the corporatization of American medicine as follows:

Me: Do you have a doctor?

Audience Member: Yes.

Me: How many patients does your doctor see each day?

Usually the response is that the person doesn't know or says something like "lots." When asked to be more specific as to numbers, it is rare that the respondent has any idea at all how many patients the doctor sees.

Today the primary care doctor most of us see when we

go in for a regular appointment is most likely employed by a large corporation. For our grandparents, the doctor was almost always self-employed. The doctor would finish medical school, come to town, and, as they say, "hang up his shingle" and go into practice. Today that kind of practice is almost nonexistent. Because it requires a lot of money to open a medical practice— and few are the doctors who could conceivably afford that—today's primary care physician is most often the employee of a large corporation.

The primary care doctor may be employed by a for-profit corporation or a not-for-profit corporation—that distinction makes little difference. As the employee of a large corporation, the first responsibility of the primary care physician is to provide the corporation a return on its investment in his salary. The physician just entering practice will usually be guaranteed an income for a period of up to two years. At the end of that time, the doctor has to be earning enough money to pay his own way plus something extra or in all likelihood he will be unemployed.

To accomplish paying his own way, a primary care physician almost anywhere in the United States today must build and maintain what's called a "patient panel" of not less than 3,000 patients. Why 3,000 patients? Because it requires that kind of a panel to generate an average of 25 to 30 office visits each day. And that's how many patients the primary

The American System:
Not About Health and Wellness

care physician is expected to see.

What this means is that a patient going in to see a primary care doctor today will have an average of six to maybe 10 minutes of time with the doctor. With increasing frequency, the patient doesn't even see the a physician. The patient sees a licensed nurse practitioner or a physician's assistant. These people are paid substantially less than the doctor because their time is considered less valuable. Fundamentally they are trained to handle many if not most routine patient visits and to triage patients to determine if they really need to see the doctor. (The term "triage" comes from the battlefield. There, when wounded soldiers arrive at the medical station, it is necessary to determine one of three things: Will the patient die regardless of what is done? Will the patient survive even though nothing is done immediately? Can the patient survive with immediate attention?)

So back to your visit to the doctor: you'll most likely be triaged and might or might not get to see the doctor. Either way, the relationship between the doctor and the patient has been transformed from what it used to be. The primary care physician's first responsibility to her employer is to generate income, which is done through ordering and referring the patient on to appropriate "specialists" who are themselves employees of the same corporation that employs the primary care doctor. Since most patients are, as I argued above, "functionally medically illiterate,"—they accept the doctor's recommendations without question.

As a result, what we have today is what I call "hamster medicine." The patient and the doctor together run around and around the cage but nobody really gets anywhere. Primary care medicine has become largely a revolving door through which patients quickly leave the doctor's office and quickly return again and again and again. The amateur patient comes in unprepared to clearly and fully explain the reasons for the visit or to understand whatever the doctor may try to teach. The doctor, in turn, is under the constant pressure of time to see more and more patients each day and thereby to spend less and less time with each one. Finally, although this may be cynical, I suggest that when all is said and done, it's all about the money.

Stepping Off the Hamster Wheel

The Professional Patient, unlike the amateur patient, understands the economic position of the primary care physician: in addition to carrying for the patient, the doctor is responsible for generating revenue for his employer. The Professional Patient also understands that the primary care doctor has only a very brief period of time in which to make a diagnosis and determine a course of action. Thus, the Professional Patient understands that time with the doctor

The American System:
Not About Health and Wellness

is at a premium and that if any real benefit is to be derived from that time, the patient has a responsibility to come into the visit well prepared.

Generally doctors appreciate Professional Patients. They appreciate patients who come in knowledgeable and prepared for their visit. They appreciate patients who come in ready to listen and to follow the instructions they are given and to seek a second opinion (more on this in Chapter 10) when they have reason to question their doctor's recommendations or to feel more secure when following them. They appreciate patients who can describe their symptoms accurately (remember "smart-ass" George from Chapter 6?).

The Skinny on Scans

Because of the fact that primary care physicians are encouraged to refer patients for tests, it has been well established that unnecessary tests and surgeries have been ordered and performed without there being a sound medical reason for doing them—but merely because they are necessary to achieve an adequate return on investment.[23]

---

2   http://www.webmd.com/news/20060519/needless-medical-tests-costly-risky?page=2

3   According to the Journal of the American College of Radiology, Vol. 5, Issue 12, pp. 1206-1209,the majority of Medicare private-office CT scans are done in facilities owned by radiologists. However, non-radiologist physicians are acquiring or leasing CT scanners in increasing numbers, and the growth trend is much more rapid among them than it is among radiologists (85 percent among radiologists from 2001 to 2006, compared with 263 percent among non-radiologists). As a result, non-radiologists'

In all fairness to the medical community it must also be noted that patients themselves are often at fault for the overuse of scans and other medical procedures. To a large degree because patients do not have, as they say, "any skin in the game" (do not have to pay for medical procedures), they demand that their doctors order them. Then doctors, in an effort to keep their patient happy and because the economics of things support the decision, order the procedures.

Consider, for example, the question of scans. Radio and television and newspapers present, on a daily basis, ads encouraging people to have a wide variety of scans. They tell us that scans can identify heart disease and cancer or that, in the absence of detecting those conditions, they can reassure us that we are healthy. Heart scans are the most commonly done. Other organs can be scanned, and frequently the whole body is scanned. There's a lot of money to be made in scanning people. Unfortunately, there is very little scientific basis for the scanning of large populations. The federal Food and Drug Administration says that people should seek scans only under the following conditions:

- When the test is for a particular disease or condition, rather than for just anything that can be found,

---

market share has increased considerably. At a time when both cost containment and reduction in radiation exposure are urgent priorities, the self-referral opportunities resulting from this trend should be of concern to payers and policymakers.

The American System:
Not About Health and Wellness

- When the test is for a disease or condition that is curable or manageable if found early enough but life threatening by the time symptoms arise,

- When the test can find that disease or condition early enough to be curable or manageable,

- When the test doesn't reveal too many findings that resemble a disease or condition that in reality would not hurt you,

- When the test doesn't miss too many cases of the disease or condition,

- When the test itself doesn't harm you significantly, and

- When the treatment for the disease or condition doesn't cause more harm than the disease or condition itself.

Remember in Chapter 5 when I talked about being diagnosed with emphysema even though I had quit smoking years earlier? I was showing a symptom—unusual shortness of breath. In that situation, the pulmonary function test was clearly appropriate because the test revealed that my shortness of breath could reasonably be attributed to my history of smoking and the subsequent damage to my lungs. Testing, especially given the very sophisticated technologies that we have today, is a valuable tool for doctors to use. Unfortunately, in a system driven to maximize profit, and given the high cost of devices such as CT scanners and MRI machines, the temptation to use these devices inappropriately is very strong. Thus we find organizations like the American Heart Association and the American Cancer Association and others issuing warnings about the inappropriate use of testing.

As a general rule, scanning should be done only when you are symptomatic for a potential condition that could be revealed by a scan or when you, by reason of age, gender, and family history, can be reasonably judged to be at higher risk for a particular condition.

The Money Business

Another characteristic of a Professional Patient is that she understands how medical care is paid for, and she can evaluate when a charge is reasonable and appropriate. The way in which medical services are paid for has undergone extensive changes just within the lifetimes of many of today's patients.

A similar situation has developed with regard to medical care. Few people today remember that as recently as 60 years ago, prior to the development of health care insurance and

The American System:
Not About Health and Wellness

programs like Medicare and Medicaid, the patient and the doctor were in a strictly one-to-one business relationship. When the patient was sick or injured, she went to the doctor. The doctor provided care in exchange for which the doctor was to be paid. If the patient could not pay with money, she paid with barter. If the patient could not even offer a barter, the doctor had a professional obligation to provide the care anyway. In this situation, though, there was very little that the doctor could do medically speaking in treating his patients, and almost nothing that would require the payment of large sums of money.

Then, after World War II, as medical knowledge and technology took huge leaps forward, it became possible for a medical treatment to cost ruinous sums, far beyond the

That Guy Nurse

ability of most people to pay. For this and other reasons, we entered into the age of both private and government health care insurance. The emergence of medical insurance has had a great many consequences for the practice of medicine, some good and some terrible. Many of them have been discussed elsewhere in this book. In the following case, we confront a typical example of the law of unintended consequences.

Cancel that Colonoscopy

Following a recent presentation, a member of the audience approached me. He was clearly angry. It seems his doctor had told him that he needed a colonoscopy. But he was outraged because his employer informed him that it was not covered as part of his health benefit. Because of this, he refused to have the procedure. In his opinion, paying for medical care was supposed to be done by his employer. He had no memory of or appreciation for the fact that throughout almost all of medical history, doctors and patients have lived in a one-to-one business relationship. The doctor provided a service. The patient paid for the service.

I was tempted to ask if, when he had the oil changed on his car, he expected somebody to pay for that. If, when he took his boat into the dealer for regular maintenance, he expected somebody to pay for that. Then I was tempted to ask why he expected somebody else to pay for his medical maintenance. But I realized that to ask these questions would be pointless. There is a pervasive attitude of entitlement regarding medical care. Just like the employees who expected to receive a gain-sharing check even though the employer had not made any money, amateur patients, without thinking about it, expect somebody else to pay for their medical care. This feeling is so deeply held by many people that they refuse to seek treatment even in the face of what could be life-threatening conditions.

This is not to suggest that all medical care should be paid for by the patient. In an age when treatments can cost thousands, tens of thousands, and even hundreds of thousands of dollars, that expectation is clearly unreasonable. At the same time, this is not to suggest that all medical care should be paid for by society, *particularly* for patients who have knowingly created their own medical problems. In Part IV, "A Vision for the Future of Medical Practice in the U.S.," I'll discuss the question of how medical care should be paid for.

Consumer-Based Health Care—Boon or Boondoggle?

There is a current movement among employers to move into providing their employees what is called "consumer-based health care." This movement is based on the thought that people are demanding "frivolous" medical care. It is argued that if patients have to pay for their medical care, they will be much more careful and cost conscious before they ask for that care. Therefore, a growing number of employers are now requiring that their employees pay up to $4,000 or more out of pocket. If and when their medical costs exceed that amount, the employer then picks up the balance. In some cases, the employer provides a tax-sheltered "health savings plan" to assist the employee. Basic to this movement is the idea that the employee must pay out of pocket for initial access to the medical system

Consumer-based health care faces two distinct problems. First, it is unclear that the patient should be held responsible for "frivolous" medical care. A patient may ask the doctor to authorize a test or procedure knowing that it will be paid for by his employer, but if the doctor agrees to provide that test or procedure in the absence of good medical reasons for doing it, it does not seem appropriate to blame the patient. The doctor, however, may order the requested test or procedure merely on the grounds that one of his responsibilities is to generate revenue for his employer, in which case the employer who does not have a "health savings plan" has to bear the cost and watch his premiums go up.

Second, unless the patient is a professional one, there is ample evidence to indicate that he will not seek medical care

The American System:
Not About Health and Wellness

in less-than-serious situations if he'll have to pay that care out of pocket. Evidence of this is that following the 2008 economic "crash," hospitals and clinics across the country reported that fewer people were seeking medical care. As a result, medical staffs were laid off in order to preserve profits. It is unlikely that the crash created a rash of "health" around the country. It is, however, reasonable to believe that paying for medical care out of pocket is not high on the priority list of the average citizen, the amateur patient.

The cost of medical care is one of the greatest problems facing the United States today. The Professional Patient, though, understands her own situation in relation to those costs and is able to accurately judge the relative costs and benefits of needed or recommended medical care.

notes:

_____

_____

_____

_____

_____

_____

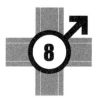

Hospitals Can Be Hazardous
to Your Health!

Almost everybody at one time or another will be a hospital patient. Almost everybody at one time or another will have a family member who is a hospital patient. Almost everybody at one time or another will have a close friend who is a hospital patient. The Professional Patient understands how hospitals work and also understands that hospitals can be very dangerous places—in fact, hazardous to your health. For this and for many other reasons, and this is one of the most important points of this book: **the patient must be in charge.**

Not the Best of All Possible Worlds

The people who work in hospitals and who have direct contact with patients are there to help. They have been educated and trained in their various roles. There are physicians. There are nurses, nursing assistants, physical therapists, phlebotomists (the Draculas who come to get your blood), radiology technicians, respiratory therapists, nutritionists, housekeepers, and a long list of other caregivers. In the best of all possible worlds, each of these people would do his or her job in a manner fully coordinated with and supportive of the work of each of the others. In the best of all possible worlds, none of these people would be rushed, stressed, or distracted.[1]

We do not, however, live in the best of all possible worlds. This is particularly important to realize in the case of the hospital. In the hospital, each and every person involved in patient care holds lives in their hands. These caregivers have the capacity either to cure or to kill.

In 2009, 99,000 Americans died of infections that they acquired while they were in a hospital.[2] Another 195,000 Americans died because of mistakes made during hospital care. For all of the miracles of surgery and healing that occur in America's hospitals, they remain very dangerous places. The Professional Patient realizes this and responds appropriately. Hospitals across the country are trying as hard as they can to bring these infections and accidents under

---

1   An important feature of recently enacted medical reform is the concept of "patient-centered medical homes" in which every patient is served by a team of caregivers working in a fully coordinated manner.

2   The Center for Disease Control reports that in 2009, 99,000 patients acquired an infection in the hospital (nosocomial infection). More than two-and-a-half million patients acquired such an infection and more than 70 percent of those infections were resistant to at least one antibiotic. Annual cost: four to five billion dollars.

some sort of control, but it will be long time before patients are out of danger.

To illustrate how dangerous life can be for the hospital patient, consider the following scenario:

The Floor Nursing Tango

I am working the day shift on the cardiac floor. My shift starts at 8 a.m., but I am at the hospital at 7 a.m. because before I can begin working with my patients, I need to know everything I can about them. So the first thing I have to do is take a report on each of the patients who has been assigned to me for this shift. The nurses on the night shift have left a tape recorded report on each patient's general condition, on any new orders that were received during the night, and on any other incidents that would be relevant to the patient's needs during the day shift. I take notes on each of my patients.

The odds are very good that one or two of my patients were admitted after my last shift. Therefore, I need to do a thorough review of each patient's history; that means going through their charts to learn why they were admitted, who their doctors are, and any relevant past history and to study any notes made on their charts by doctors or other staff upon their admission. Then and only then am I ready to begin my day.

The first event of the day is usually the eight a.m. medication pass. All over the country at eight a.m., tens of thousands of nurses are doing the same thing: getting ready to deliver the ordered medications to their patients. On an average shift, I will have four or five patients assigned to my care. Two of them are recovering from open heart surgery. Two had angioplasties yesterday and will probably be discharged today. The fifth patient was brought in last night with a suspected heart attack. He is currently being evaluated.

My five patients will, collectively, receive anywhere from 12 to 20 different medications at eight a.m. There will be pain medications, blood pressure medications, antibiotics, medications to control and regulate heartbeat, and stool softeners. Two patients are diabetic, and there are medications for their diabetes. One patient is receiving an anti-anxiety medication. The computer gives me a printout for each patient of the medications he or she is to receive at eight a.m. I go to a medication dispensing machine in the nursing station. I enter each patient's identifying code into the computer and drawers open, each containing one or more of that patient's medications. Each drawer may contain four or five different medications. They may be the same medication in different doses or completely different medications.

That Guy Nurse

As the drawers containing my patients' meds open, I withdraw a med from each drawer and place it in a small paper cup that I have prepared with the patient's room number and name printed on the side. Since I have five patients, there are five cups sitting on the counter in front of me. Now just imagine how many opportunities there are for me to make an error. As I write this, hospitals are developing new protocols intended to reduce medication errors. It is still necessary for the Professional Patient to take steps to reduce danger. When patient and nurse realize and grasp the idea the they are partners in a joint effort to be safe, then things will really improve.

Now also realize that while I am gathering together my medications, four or five other nurses are standing next to me, each retrieving the medications for their patients and dropping them into the paper cups that they have prepared. Now the opportunities for error are multiplied, and errors do get made.

As I am retrieving the medications for my patients, a doctor is waiting impatiently at the nursing station to discuss some new orders for one of his patients. The nursing assistant who is working with me tells me that one of my patients is having chest pain. Two family members of another patient are waiting impatiently to discuss with me why they feel that their dad has not received the quality of care that they expect.

Hospitals Can Be Hazardous to Your Health

Finally, the charge nurse has just let me know that I'm going to take in a new admission who will be arriving in about 30 minutes. This situation is rife with opportunities for error.

Mixed Heparin: The Story of an Error

It's two o'clock in the afternoon. I began working for day shift on the cardiac floor at 7 a.m. One of the nurses scheduled for the second shift has called in sick. The charge nurse puts out the call for somebody willing to work a double. Nobody responds. I'm the only guy on the day shift, and I am 61 years old. That means I don't have any children at home. And so all eyes turn toward me. Once again, I agree to work the double.

The way things work out, I don't get to keep any of the patients I had during the day. They had already been assigned to another nurse on second shift. And so I sit down and go through the tape recorded report on five new patients. Luckily, the shift goes fairly easily with no major emergencies or distractions. I do have two patients, both males, who had angioplasties during the day. They are in room 252. They are each on an I.V. solution designed to prevent blood clots. It's called heparin. The thing about heparin is that it has a very powerful effect, and therefore patients who are receiving heparin intravenously must have their blood checked regularly to make sure that it is neither too thin nor not thin enough.

An ongoing problem on the floor is that there are 12 cardiologists who can send patients to this unit. And no two of them share the same heparin protocol, that is, the schedule under which they want their patients' coagulation time (PT) checked. We nurses had formed a committee about a year ago to try and convince the cardiologists to adopt the same heparin protocol. We thought we had succeeded. But then, within a matter of weeks, each cardiologist began writing amendments. So it was that I had two patients in the same room on different heparin protocols.

It's now 11:15 p.m. A call comes from the laboratory giving me the PT values on the patient in room 252, bed 2. I take the laboratory report to the patient's chart to find out what the heparin protocol requires. Sometimes the heparin rate of drip has to be increased and sometimes decreased. In this case, I was supposed to increase the rate of the heparin drip. The patients' room is dark and I don't want to wake them up. I quietly slip into the room, go to the intravenous pump hanging at the bedside, and adjust the drip rate. I quietly return to the hallway and immediately realize that I have adjusted the drip rate on the wrong patient. Somewhat less quietly I return to the room and repair the error.

The rules of the floor require that when an error like this

is made, it must be reported. I dutifully fill out an error slip. It's important to realize that no damage was done in this case. The error was fixed before it had any effect on either patient. Nonetheless, the next day I'm called to see the manager to explain how I made the error. I pointed out that I've worked a double, and that I had been working for nearly 17 hours. I pointed out that there were two patients in room 252 and that each was on a different heparin protocol. It was made clear to me that this kind of error was not acceptable and that I would have to be more careful. A note was made on my personnel record.

Mistakes Are Made

The simple fact is that floor nursing is a high-stress job. And it is almost impossible not to make mistakes. Consider just the medications. These are not M&Ms or Hershey kisses. These are medications that can heal or, given inappropriately, kill.

My employer, the hospital, is constantly pressured by the need to make a profit. In addition, the people who pay for medical care, the private insurance companies or the government, place constant pressure on my employer to reduce costs. Thus, as the provision of medical care has become ever more complex and high tech, and as patients generally come in sicker and are sent home sooner, the people who must provide the care are under increasing pressure to achieve maximum efficiency. Meanwhile the nurse is expected to present a warm and caring face to the patient and family. She must present a respectful and professional face to the doctors. She must provide ongoing support to her peers on the nursing team. It all adds up to stress.

One of the results of these competing goals—providing medical care of the highest quality at the lowest possible cost—is that mistakes are made. The Professional Patient is aware of this and takes every possible precaution to see that he is not the victim of one of these mistakes.

The hospital administration stated that all errors should be reported. No disciplinary action would follow. The purpose for reporting errors was to ensure that they did not happen again. However, it was common knowledge among the nursing staff that reporting errors could and did lead to some very unpleasant consequences. Thus, it was also common knowledge that some errors were never reported. A nurse who did not report an error could feel quite secure that no other nurse would make a report. This was a matter of mutual self-protection.

Consider another example of how hospitals can be dangerous to your health. Most patients will have two or more doctors involved in their inpatient care. In the best of al possible worlds, every doctor involved in a patient's care would be in perfect communication with each of the others. In the real world, however, this kind of communication is, although not rare, far from common. Two or more doctors may be writing medication orders on a patient. Each is writing orders for a problem: irregular heart beat, diabetes, constipation, fever, pain, and on and on. Ideally each doctor would consult the list of current medications being taken by the patient. Yeah! No, the way it really works is that the nurse caring for a patient must, when a new medication is ordered, consult a chart to determine whether the new medication is compatible with all current medications. Too often there is a conflict(s), and the nurse has to reach the prescribing doctor to have him change his order.

One more time: **hospitals are dangerous places**. Modern medicine is very complex. Physicians tend to want to do things their own way. In an effort to reduce costs, staff is kept at minimum levels. Ironically, this combination of circumstances contributes to the danger of the errors that are such a significant factor in the high levels of mortality experienced in America's hospitals

> ## "Doctor, I have something to tell you."
>
> Early in my nursing career, I received an order for a new medication for one of my patients. I checked the new med against those already ordered. I discovered that new research strongly indicated that the new med should not be administered in the ordered dose while my patient was on one of his current meds. I phoned the doctor with this information. His response (paraphrased for the more delicate readers): "What the Hell! Are you trying to tell me how to practice medicine? I don't give a ___ what you think. I am the doctor and I will write the orders I want. Don't ever call me with this kind of s**t again!"

Precautions You Can Take

First, the Professional Patient arranges that unless she is fully alert and competent to direct her own care, somebody—a friend or family member surrogate—will be present in the room at all times to provide that direction and protection.

Every caregiver, nurse or technician, who enters the room will be asked to identify themselves, to identify the patient, and to state the purpose of their visit. That way we know that everyone is singing from the same page of the hymn book. Normally this is done as a matter of course, but if the caregiver does not do these things, the patient or the patient's surrogate will ensure that they are done.

This is important, because today's hospital worker is almost always dealing with high levels of daily stress. First, patients come and go more quickly. As an example, consider the fact that as recently as 25 years ago, a mother, following delivery of her baby, would spend a week in the hospital. Today she may spend two days, if that. Thus, it is difficult for nurses and other hospital staff to come to know their patients well. Second, medications are more numerous and more potent. They can cure or kill depending on whether or not the nurse remembers the 5R's: to give the Right medication to the Right patient in the Right dose at the Right time and by the Right method. There are more and more technical specialists entering patient rooms: phlebotomists, physical therapists, occupational therapists, radiology technicians, nutritionists, and the list goes on and on. As said above, the plain fact is that up to 195,000 patients die each year because someone in the hospital made a mistake. Thousands of others are damaged by errors that can and do cause permanent harm but that do not kill. And one of the biggest mistakes lies in the misidentification of the patient.

Second, nobody—doctor, caregiver, friend, or family member—will have any physical contact with the patient until and unless they have washed their hands. Most hospital rooms today have a canister of hand cleanser located just inside the door. It must be used. One of the major causes for tens of thousands of patients dying each year from hospital-acquired infections is that people forget to wash their hands thoroughly. And that includes doctors as well as caregivers, family members, and other visitors.

Patients, family, and friends are often afraid to challenge hospital staff. Professional Patients have the courage and the assertiveness to do just that. Remember, this is a partnership in which the patient partner is not only the equal of the others but is and must always be in charge.

Third, the Professional Patient or her surrogate will ask the nurse delivering medications to identify each medication and to match it with the computerized printout of the schedule and medications that are to be given. If medications come pre-packaged, the ID on the package must be confirmed.

Fourth, nobody—no doctor, no nurse, no technician—will touch a patient with a stethoscope until the stethoscope has been, within sight, wiped down with an alcohol or other antiseptic wipe. After all, you don't know where that stethoscope was five minutes ago.

None of this will make the Professional Patient or his surrogates very popular with the staff. They may be known that the nursing station as "the difficult patient in 247." But that's okay. Ultimately the only thing that makes any difference is that patients regain their health and leave the hospital better than they were when they came in.

Patients and family members are in a difficult position. Just as many people will not ask their doctor for a second opinion for fear that the doctor will think they do not trust him them or that the doctor will not like them (see Chapter 10 for more on the second opinion), patients and family members are often reluctant to question nurses and other caregivers. Yet this can and must be done. A good way to do it is to precede the request by saying, for example, "I know how busy and stressful your life can be. But I know, too, that even very professional people can make mistakes. So I hope you won't mind if I . . . (then state your question or request here)."

Perhaps if patients, in demanding the kind of care that they should be receiving, speak loudly enough, the system may change and everybody will benefit.

What's Up with Those Nurses?

It's eight o'clock in the evening. You and the rest of the family have come to visit grandma. She's a patient on the nursing floor after surgery. As you step off the elevator, you notice four nurses sitting at the nursing station eating cookies and talking. You think to yourself, "Is that all they've got to do?" I have often heard that sentiment expressed by people who think that the nurses ought to be taking care of their patients and not just sitting around or that nursing is a pretty cushy job.

Every once in awhile it is true that that group of nurses has, for a moment, nothing better to do than relax. But believe me, as a nurse, I treasure those occasional moments when my patients are resting quietly, there are no doctors roaming the floor, the supper trays have all been collected and sent back to the kitchen, my charting is up to date, and the printer from the laboratory that is constantly typing out lab reports—most of which require that I call a doctor and get new orders—is sitting silently in the corner. In the course of a normal shift, those few moments are precious.

Think of it this way. You go to visit the neighborhood fire station. A few of the firefighters are cleaning an engine. Others are fixing a piece of equipment. But a number of them are sitting in the lounge watching TV and playing cribbage. You think to yourself, "Boy, are we overstaffed with firefighters." No, given the nature of their work, I don't think we fault them for grabbing some time just to relax. It's pretty much the same way with nursing. Nursing and a few other professions can properly be described as, "hours of sheer boredom punctuated by moments of stark terror." In nursing, there are rarely hours of boredom but there are moments of stark terror: unanticipated and unanticipatable moments when a patient's life hangs in the balance and everything depends upon the nurse knowing exactly what to do and doing it.

A further complication in the nurse's life is the result of management's effort to ensure that the hospital is profitable. Staffing levels are kept as low as possible. Combine that fact with the realization that medical technology and pharmaceutical developments have made the tasks of the nurse incredibly more complex than they were just a few decades ago. Finally, realize that, because of the push to generate profit, the people occupying patient beds are rarely healthy and well. They are sick. They are very sick. The minute they are barely well enough to be discharged, they are gone.

I treasure those occasions in which, for just a few minutes, I can sit quietly and discuss this weekend's Packer game or what a pain the new cardiologist is. But in the back of my mind, on the edge of my consciousness, is the thought that a patient call light can come on at any moment, dragging me back into the reality that the people I am caring for need me.

Another Unanticipated Consequence

Just a few decades ago, children were not allowed to visit patients in their rooms. The children themselves were at risk for infection, and they created a risk of infecting the patient. Then hospitals decided to become family friendly, part of the growing competition among hospitals. As a result, entire families now come trooping into patient rooms.

People generally think of hospitals is being antiseptically clean. Nothing could be farther from the truth. The housekeeping staff and the staff working on the floor do their best to keep things clean. But at the same time, all kinds of people come onto the floor and into patient rooms. Those people bring with them all kinds of things that are not clean. They bring gifts, they bring flowers. Heck, they bring themselves—and what's on the bottoms of their shoes? And the patients they are visiting are sick. Their immune systems are compromised. Often they have large incisions that are open invitations for infection.

A Baby's Kiss (of Death?)

Grandma is just two days out of open heart surgery. She has a long incision down the middle of her chest. It has been carefully dressed with bandages to protect it from infectious organisms. Then the family arrives. The chances are very good that when they arrive, the nurse is away at other duties. Even if the nurse is present in the room, it can be difficult trying to tell the family what they can or should not do. And so the family insists that the baby give grandma a kiss. The baby is picked up and, in the process of kissing grandma, is rubbed across grandma's chest. Far too often, Grandma develops an infection and then Grandma dies after a successful surgery.

Hospitals Can Be Hazardous to Your Health

It always fascinates me when the visitors include a child. Children get bored quickly. And so it often happens that the parents tell that child to simply be quiet and play. And where does the child play? On the floor, naturally. It's a bright shiny floor. It looks clean and freshly waxed. But what the family doesn't know is that 30 minutes before they arrived, grandma needed to go to the bathroom. With the help of a nursing assistant, we walked her from her bed to the bathroom. But on the way, grandma peed on the floor. My nursing assistant got a towel and wiped it up. She calls housekeeping, but they haven't arrived yet. Essentially the child is playing in grandma's pee.

Back to the point made above. You, if you are the patient, or if somebody you care about is the patient, must be in charge. All of the people working in the medical system are there to help. Think of them as your partners. Everyone in the system needs to work together. Patients and families and friends, together with doctors and nurses and all of the other members of the medical team, must, at all times, be partners working together to achieve the end that everybody wants. Partnership requires that all the partners participate in achieving the outcome, which is the purpose of the partnership.

The patient is, and I will keep on repeating this, the senior partner.

That Guy Nurse

Again, as was pointed out in Chapter 6, the patient can and must be the CEO of his own life. All of the other people in the partnership, which is the medical team, are there for one and only one purpose, one goal: to restore the patient to health.

notes:

_____

_____

_____

_____

_____

_____

_____

_____

_____

_____

_____

_____

Hospitals Can Be Hazardous to Your Health

Choosing A Physician:
Your Doctor's Job Description

In the modern world of medicine, the vision of the family doctor, the old family friend who made house calls and sat by the bedside of the sick child, is a legend of the past. The modern physician, the primary care doctor, is located in a clinic, surrounded by nurses and assistants and accountants, faced with seeing 25 to 30 patients a day. He can spend an average of only six to 10 minutes with each patient. He is swamped with paperwork. He no longer makes visits to his patients who are in the hospital. That duty has been assigned to a new breed of physician, the "hospitalist." This is hamster medicine. The wheel goes round and round, but it does not go anywhere. The result is that primary care medicine resembles a revolving door. Patients come and go round and round through the door, but it is rare that they make progress toward improved health or a longer life.

As our medical knowledge about prevention, early

detection, medications, and treatments has grown, the ability of the system to pass that information through to patients has correspondingly shrunk. Thus we are a nation of people who are medically illiterate.

Modern patients must begin taking matters into their own hands. Patients can no longer merely be "patient." Patients must become proactive, assertive, and even demanding when it comes to their access to medical care. One of the most important things patients can do is to make sure that their doctor is the right doctor for them. The best way to do this is to meet with and to interview doctors until the right one is found. We don't employ contractors to remodel our kitchens or bathrooms or even to roof our homes without seeking references and looking at pictures of their prior efforts and even interviewing their former clients. Why, then, do we entrust our health and even our lives to someone who is little more than a stranger?

Unless you are totally happy with and confident in your current physician, and especially if you do not currently have a physician (get one!), you should choose a clinic and then request to meet with a physician to interview him and decide if this should be your doctor. You will ask about the doctor's sense of his own strengths and weaknesses and interests, such as children, the elderly, men, women, etc. Is this a person who will be willing to spend time listening and teaching? If not, move on, seek another. Ask friends about their doctors and how they feel about their doctors. If you rely on them for help in choosing someone to re-do your kitchen, maybe you can rely on them when they recommend a doctor.

Going to the Web can be helpful in choosing a doctor. There are a number of sites that carry information about physicians and their records. Try searching for "Doctor Ratings." Dozens of sites are available. Many require a fee for search. Those that are free are often worth just about as much as they charge. You will have to judge the worth of any given site providing physician evaluations. Still, there are recourses on the Web.

Be creative... finding the right doctor can well be a matter of life and health or of death.

You are the president of your own life. You doctor is your secretary of health. Your doctor serves at your pleasure. You are and must be in charge. The time to do this is not when you are sick or injured but now. Now, when you have your health and are willing to work with your doctor, in partnership, to stay healthy. The interview is the foundation of a medical partnership, and it will benefit both your and your doctor.

A Medical Parable

Once upon a time across the nation automobiles by the

Choosing A Physician: Your Doctor's Job Description

tens of millions began to fail

Streets and highways were littered with abandoned cars and trucks. Their engines had been destroyed for lack of oil. Their transmissions had frozen as their fluids had drained away. Many were the victims of crashes, as brake linings had worn to the point that they could no longer function. Tens of thousands of fatalities had been the result.

People by the millions did not have the financial means to repair ruined automobiles. People could not get to work, and businesses were forced to close for lack of employees. The situation seemed hopeless.

The authorities were mystified. The government had spent billions to ensure that the automobile companies could continue to produce cars. There was a massive inventory of engines, transmissions, and brake linings in auto dealerships in every state. There were inventories of millions of quarts of oil accumulating dust on dealership shelves. What happened?

Congress, of course, held hearings to discover the cause(s) of the disaster. It was discovered that hardly anyone thought to do preventive maintenance on their vehicles. People just ignored their maintenance manuals. Few understood the basic principles of the internal combustion engine or that machines of every sort require lubrication. The hearings revealed that the great majority of people drove their vehicles hard. They constantly accelerated with screeching tires and, approaching stop lights, sped up until the last minute and then jumped so hard on their brakes that their tires left black marks on the roads.

It was discovered that dealerships, realizing that there was more money to be made in selling new vehicles and repairing worn or damaged ones than in promoting preventive maintenance, rarely emphasized preventive maintenance to their customers or rewarded them when they did practice preventive maintenance.

It was concluded that the vast majority of drivers had destroyed their cars and trucks through simple ignorance. They didn't understood how their cars worked, and thus they did not know how to keep them running. In their ignorance, they didn't practice preventive maintenance. They drove their cars and trucks in ways that inevitably led to their destruction.

Finally, those who could have taught drivers how to keep their cars operating safely and reliably, those who manufactured, sold, and maintained cars, had no interest in doing so. They were in business to make money, and there was little money in keeping cars running safely and reliably.

The Doctor's Role

Once you have found your doctor, how should you use

him? For most of us, the doctor has been a kind of mechanic that one goes to when something is broken, burning, bleeding, oozing, or causing pain. That was most certainly the role of the doctor for our parents and grandparents. The Professional Patient understands that the physician can have a very different role today. The doctor today can and must be a coach and a mentor in the important business of attaining and maintaining good health. Certainly there will be situations in which one is sick or injured and requires the services of the doctor and, perhaps, the specialist, to restore health. But for the Professional Patient, those situations are the exception.

To understand the doctor's role today, think of the mechanic who works on your car. When you purchased your car, you probably read through the owner's manual. It told you how to turn on the headlights, how to open the trunk, how to tune the radio, and a hundred other little pieces of knowledge that allowed you to use your car. The manual also had a section on recommended maintenance. It gave you a chart on one side of which mileages were listed: 1000 miles, 3000 miles, 5000 miles 20,000 miles. Reading across the chart from each of those mileage intervals were the specific things that must be done to keep the car running and running safely. You were instructed as to when to change the oil, change the transmission fluid, rotate the tires, tune the engine, and perform dozens of other tasks, all of which were required to keep your car "healthy."

This is called "preventive maintenance." Most likely you paid attention to the advice in the owner's manual. After all, you have a big investment in the car and you count on it to get you reliably and safely to work, to the store, and to the family vacation. Now realize that you and your car share at least one thing in common: you both require good preventive maintenance.

Perhaps the most important service your secretary of health can provide is that of giving you your personal owner's manual. This is the most basic part of your partnership. Your contribution? Information about your family's medical history and accurate information about your lifestyle. The Professional Patient researches family medical history, at least that of mother and father, aunts and uncles, cousins, brothers and sisters, and his own.

In Chapter 6 it was pointed out that a family medical history can provide insight into the medical problems most likely to affect each of us. Keep in mind, though, that a person's medical history identifies tendencies, not destiny. Because of that, knowledge of family history and lifestyle allows the doctor to prescribe those tests that can detect potentially serious problems early, and, more fortunately, can

Choosing A Physician: Your Doctor's Job Description

teach his patients how to take the steps necessary to prevent those problems from ever occurring or to identify problems before they become serious. This is preventive maintenance combined with early testing and diagnosis.

There's one big problem with early testing and diagnosis: getting it done! It's not likely when we take our car in for routine maintenance that we're going to be told that our car is terminal. And even if we get that terrible message, we can always get another car. It's not quite that way with medical preventive maintenance. If the tests reveal that something is wrong, our options are not as simple as installing a new muffler or buying a new set of tires. As a result, we tend to be fearful of medical tests. And a common response to the fear is not to have any.

During my 23 years working in hospice as a volunteer and as a nurse, I found that many if not most, of the patients I cared for as they were dying either did not understand the concept of early testing and diagnosis or were simply afraid to take the tests that could have revealed their cancer before it became lethal. In that sense, and for that reason, they were dying unnecessarily.

Likewise, on the cardiac floor, many of my patients,

generally men but not always, were there because they had experienced a heart attack and were now dying of the subsequent heart disease. As we talked about their situation, they revealed that prior to the heart attack, there had been months and even years of recurrent episodes of chest pain accompanied by a light sweat or maybe pain in the jaw or tingling in the fingers on the left hand. These episodes had been dismissed as being the products of last night's pizza or stress at work or some other easily ignored condition. The common the response was to take an antacid tablet. But almost always there was some fear that these were the symptoms of a heart attack. That was too frightening a prospect to face, and so the symptoms were wished away. Again, there is an old saying, "Denial ain't just a river in Egypt."

Time and time again people I have cared for, for reasons of fear and ignorance and sometimes because of lack of money, did not seek the services of a doctor. When, finally, their symptoms of chest pain, of unusual bleeding, of fatigue (this could be a long list) became so serious that they had no choice but to see a doctor, it was too late. "I'm sorry, Bill. You had a heart attack. We're not going to let you die, but you're going to spend the rest of your life on medications and, I'm sorry, but never again are you going to do most of the things that you love." Or, "Mary, I'm sorry to have to tell

Choosing A Physician: Your Doctor's Job Description

you that you have a cancer. It has metastasized. It is spread throughout your body and there's nothing we can do. I'm going to refer you to hospice."

These are terrible situations, but they are repeated hundreds of thousands of times every year. Why? We are amateurs in a world that demands that we become professionals.

Committing oneself to a schedule of preventive maintenance requires courage. Unlike simply waiting until things go wrong before seeing a doctor, preventive maintenance requires that we acknowledge the possibility of our own mortality. We cannot escape our mortality, but we can reduce the chance of early death. Professional Patients have the courage to practice prevention and early diagnosis. And it does take courage in the face of what is almost an instinct to live with denial.

So, you go to your doctor with all the information you can gather on your family's medical history.[1] He looks at that information. He knows your age and your gender and he begins to formulate your personal maintenance schedule. There are a lot of cardiac problems in your family. You are in your 40s. Your doctor suggests that you will come into the office at least once a year for a blood pressure check

---

1   The most common reason why adoptive children are going into the courts to seek information about their birth parents is their need for information about family medical history.

and a cholesterol test. He suggests that you have an EKG every four years, and he orders a cardiac stress test (the dreaded treadmill) every four years. He makes sure that you understand the signs and symptoms of heart disease. He asks you to promise that you will call him if you think that anything may be going wrong.

There is almost no reason to die from heart disease or a heart attack. And the reason why heart disease is the number one taker of life in the United States is that people are not Professional Patients. They do not understand the vital importance of preventive care or of health-promoting life choices.

Your doctor looks at your family medical history and sees that cancer is a common occurrence. He suggests that you have (depending on gender) a PAP test, a mammogram, a prostate-specific antigen test, a colonoscopy, or any of a number of other tests that can detect potentially lethal conditions before they become fatal. Although cancer is the second leading cause of death in the United States, there are very few cancers that are neither preventable nor detectable before they become lethal. It all depends on the Professional Patient, in partnership with a doctor, to practice preventive maintenance and to implement the plan provided by their doctor.

Choosing A Physician: Your Doctor's Job Description

As I discussed in more detail in Chapter 7, although preventive maintenance is a key to living long and dying healthy, the Professional Patient also realizes that the medical system has an inherent bias toward ordering tests that may be unnecessary but that do generate income. Therefore, the Professional Patient, when asked to undergo any kind of medical test, asks her doctor why test is indicated, what the test is likely to reveal, what the dangers of the test may be, and what the frequency of false positives that test has.[2]

You and your doctor are a team. You are a team of professionals. You are the captain. Like any other team, you have a goal. The goal is that you'll be healthy. Like any other team, your team, if it is to be successful, requires teamwork and cooperation. To abuse an old metaphor, your team is only as strong as its weakest member. If your doctor is not knowledgeable, conscientious, and caring, she cannot do you much good. If you are not likewise knowledgeable, conscientious, and caring, your doctor cannot do you much good.

---

2   The concept of false positives is little understood. If a test has a high number of false positives, each of which may require subsequent tests and or treatments that may be unnecessary or even dangerous, the Professional Patient has to make a decision. But that is what professionals do. Often there are alternative tests to the one a doctor may recommend. The Professional Patient asks if there are alternatives and what the virtues of those alternatives may be.

That Guy Nurse

notes:

_____

_____

_____

_____

_____

_____

_____

_____

_____

_____

_____

_____

_____

_____

_____

_____

Choosing A Physician: Your Doctor's Job Description

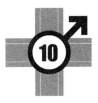

The Second Opinion:
Don't Proceed Without It

The Professional Patient almost always seeks a second medical opinion. This is especially true in the case of a proposed surgery or any other medical procedure that seems to be in any sense out of the ordinary. Why is a second opinion so important? For two reasons. First, the diagnosis that leads to a recommended course of treatment—surgical or pharmaceutical or therapeutic—always contains an element of guesswork. Second, almost all recommended treatments or tests have an element of risk.

The physician examines the body of information available regarding your condition. She examines your initial complaint and your history and current information, such as temperature, blood pressure, the results of blood tests, and the results of scans such as CT and MRI scans. Using all of this information, she arrives at a diagnosis.

In most cases, the presenting information is adequate to support a diagnosis with near certainty. But in a significant number of cases, especially those where the diagnosis is of a condition that is potentially life threatening, the connection between data and diagnosis may be far from close, and the recommended treatment will probably entail some risk for the patient. There are, of course, emergency situations that do not allow the time to seek a second opinion. Overall, however, the vast majority of medical diagnoses are made in situations that are not critical emergencies. In these cases, seeking a second opinion should be standard operating procedure. If needed, you might even ask for a third opinion. It is, after all, your health and life that are involved.

Consider, too, the old maxim, "If your only tool is a hammer, every problem is a nail." Surgeons tend to see surgery as the answer to the patient's problems. Other, nonsurgical specialties, therapy, pharmaceutical, etc., might well have a different answer. Note that current research suggests quite strongly that many if not most open heart surgeries did not extend the life of the patients or even reduce the likelihood of future heart attacks.[1]

Quite often patients seeking a second opinion choose to go to the Mayo Clinic, to the Cleveland Clinic, or to some other famous medical facility. They do this thinking that they

---

1   John Carey, "Is Heart Surgery Worth It?" Bloomberg Businessweek, July 18, 2005.

That Guy Nurse

will receive a better diagnosis and, if it should be necessary, better medical treatment. Unfortunately, this is far too often not the case. I like to say that if you have a medical problem that is so rare that only a few dozen other people on the planet have the same problem, you might want to go to one of these famous clinics. Why? They have probably seen most of the others already. But most of the time and for most people, a high-quality second opinion can be had without the time and expense of going to the "world-class" medical centers.

In the majority of situations, the business of diagnosis as well as treatment is not rocket science. As is the case with primary care medicine, the chief criterion of quality and success is the combination of time on task and repetition. The more time that the doctor spends with a patient, the better the outcomes of that relationship are likely to be. The more times a surgeon has performed a specific surgery, the better the outcome of that surgery is likely to be. The Professional Patient seeking medical care will always want to know that his doctor will spend the time necessary talking about what is being recommended and why it is being recommended. In the case of surgery, the Professional Patient will find out how often the surgeon has performed that surgery. The single most important factor in surgical success is the number of times the surgeon and the surgical team have performed the

The Second Opinion: Don't Proceed Without It

Two or Ten?

Some years ago my wife Rosalie and I were dining at a local restaurant. Rosalie made a gesture with her right hand and suddenly her hand froze in mid-air, and she said in a very frightened voice, "I can't see out of my right eye!" She moved her hand to cover her left eye and confirmed that she was blind on the right side.

As quickly as I could, I called a friend who was a ophthalmologist who directed me to bring her to the office immediately. Once there, he quickly diagnosed that she had a detached retina. He told her that she needed surgery at once. He informed her that he would contact a local surgeon. Then, Rosalie, being a Professional Patient, asked him, "Doctor, if you needed this surgery, who would you have do it?" His response: "I would go to Dr.Collins in Milwaukee."

With Rosalie lying on her back, her head braced between two pillows in the back seat of the car, we drove to Milwaukee. There Dr. Collins performed the surgery to reattach her retina. Checking back, I found that the local surgeon performed maybe two or three retinal reattachments per month while Dr. Collins did as many as ten each week.

operation in question.

Once a diagnosis has been given, there are often many options that must be considered regarding the best treatment. Here is where the Professional Patient should be especially alert. Both the primary doctor and the doctor from whom a second opinion is sought should be asked about alternate

That Guy Nurse

modes of treatment. It turns out that in many cases, surgery, although entailing more risk, does little more to extend the patient's life or quality of life than would aggressive pharmaceutical treatment. In addition, surgery today always entails some of the additional danger of nosocomial (hospital-acquired) infection.[2]

Terry's Story

Here is a case that illustrates the potential importance of the second opinion as well as the importance of the patient doing some independent research. The patient's name is Terry. About 10 years ago, he was diagnosed with emphysema. He had been a smoker for more than 20 years but had quit the habit 34 years ago. He was experiencing increasing shortness of breath with exertion and so underwent a pulmonary function test.

The test resulted in the diagnosis of emphysema. Smoking had destroyed so much of Terry's lungs that they were not able to transfer an adequate amount of oxygen into his blood. He ran short of breath with minimal exertion. His heart was forced to beat more rapidly in order to pass more blood through his lungs. Emphysema cannot be cured. However, the shortness of breath that is the primary symptom of

---

2   The National Institues of Health report that in 2007, approximately 95,000 to 110,000 patients died from nosocomial infections.

The Second Opinion: Don't Proceed Without It

emphysema can be treated in a variety of ways.[3]

Recently Terry was experiencing what he took to be an increasing shortness of breath. He spoke to his doctor, who recommended another pulmonary function test. The test revealed that the emphysema had worsened. Now, though, the doctor suggested that, since Terry was in his 70s, there was a possibility of cardiac insufficiency (his heart was weakening), which should also be explored. At this point, things started to get complicated.

The first recommended test was called a "cardiac calcium score." The calcium score is derived from a CT scan of the heart. The scan can reveal the presence of calcification in the coronary arteries indicating the presence of some form of blockage. It turned out that a local hospital was offering the test for only $50. Normally the test could cost $300 or $400.

Now there are two possible reasons why the hospital was doing this. It is possible that the hospital was attempting to reach out to offer the community an opportunity for early diagnosis, which could lead to patients taking appropriate preventive action to detect what could be a serious medical condition. At the same time, it is not unreasonable to suggest that this offer of a very low-cost calcium score is

---

3 Here is another situation in which the Professional Patient questions the doctor about alternative modes of treatment and their benefits, costs, and dangers. It is also a point at which one might seek a second opinion.

That Guy Nurse

just what retailers call a "loss leader." They take a loss on some products just to draw people into the store. Doctors may face pressures to refer patients for this test merely as a revenue enhancer, since many of the patients who have the test will be referred for more tests, all of which will cost a lot.[4]

Terry's calcium score indicated that there was some blockage or blockages in his coronary arteries. The test, it turned out, did not reveal the exact location or severity of the blockage(s). Thus, it was recommended that Terry have a further test. Terry's doctor suggested that he have a test called a CT angiogram. Sensing a pattern developing here, Terry did some research. Almost immediately he found two interesting pieces of information. He found that a CT angiogram involves the patient receiving the equivalent of more than 1100 chest x-rays. He also found that the American Cardiology Association was expressing concern that the procedure was being overused and that at least part of the overuse was probably based on the desire of the hospitals and physicians groups who owned the scanning equipment to achieve a better return on their investment.

Armed with this information, Terry talked to the cardiologist who was scheduled to do the procedure (the

---

4   It is interesting that within a few days of the hospital offering the $50 dollar calcium score, a nearby hospital advertised in the paper that it was offering the test for $49.95.

The Second Opinion: Don't Proceed Without It

second opinion). When asked directly if this is the procedure the cardiologist would recommend, he responded, "Well, the normal thing would be to do a nuclear stress test."

Terry chose the nuclear stress test. In this test, the patient receives an injection of a slightly radioactive substance. The heart is then exercised to maximize blood flow to the heart muscle. Subsequent scans will reveal if there are any areas of the heart that are not receiving adequate blood flow. The test showed some mild but probably age-related problems. Nothing serious.

However, when the cardiologist was unable to assess the base (bottom) of the heart, it was suggested that Terry have an echocardiogram. In an echocardiogram, sound waves are used to develop a picture of the heart, much as they are used in the sonogram that gives a picture of a baby in the uterus. Following the echocardiogram, Terry was informed that although there were some slight abnormalities, he basically had the heart of a 73-year-old man. In other words, everything was normal and no further interventions were recommended.

Without the promise of a cheap, $50 test it is unlikely that Terry would ever have embarked on this series of tests. Once started, however, the outcome was inevitable. The hospital made a lot of money, Terry learned that he was just a 73-year-old-man, and the taxpayers had another new bill to pay.

The Professional Patient understands all of this. He understands that doctors, like their employers, can offer treatments and tests that are not in the patient's best interests but that serve to enhance the revenues of both physician and hospital. When the Professional Patient goes out to buy a car, he knows that the salesman will try to load the car with accessories. When he shops for a television, he knows that the salesman will try to get him to buy the biggest and most expensive set. He knows that similar motivations also work in American medicine.

As an ironic conclusion to the above story, Terry, after receiving his results, spoke with another cardiologist, a friend. The friend commented that he would never have a cardiac scan unless he was unequivocally symptomatic. That is, unless Terry had had clear symptoms of heart disease, this doctor felt that there was no reason to have any further tests. Let's call this a third opinion, only one offered just a little too late.

The point of all of this is to say that medicine, as much as it is a matter of science, is also a human endeavor. People do make mistakes. People often have mixed motives for their actions. Unless there is a close and trusting partnership

The Second Opinion: Don't Proceed Without It

between the patient and his doctor, mistakes can be made. And when mistakes can be made, they will be made. This is Murphy's Law.

Modern technology has created many situations in which the desire for financial gain on the part of the medical establishment overrides what is good for the patient. The Professional Patient, therefore, will always be somewhat suspicious of recommended tests and procedures that are not clearly necessary.[5]

Take Your Time

As I said above, very few medical procedures, especially surgical procedures, need to be done on an emergency basis. Almost always there is time to seek a second opinion. Yet amateur patients rarely ask for one. Their concern seems to be, "The doctor will think I don't trust him" or "The doctor won't like me." Please be assured a competent and caring doctor will never resent a Professional Patient asking for a second opinion.

Here's a possible way to phrase it: "Doctor, I would really appreciate if I could have a second opinion. I have great confidence in you, but I know that it would make me

---

5   For more information on CT screening, go to this useful federal government Web site: www.fda.gov/cdrh/ct/screening.html <http://www.fda.gov/cdrh/ct/screening.html>

feel better if I could have a second opinion. I would like to speak with a doctor in another medical system, preferably in another town.

When a patient requests a second opinion, one of two things will happen. Either the doctor will agree that this is a good idea, or he will hesitate and perhaps suggest that it really isn't necessary. A truly competent and caring doctor recognizes that when a patient requests a second opinion, he is dealing with a Professional Patient. The competent and caring doctor wants the second opinion himself. He wants it for four reasons.

First, it's his way of showing off for his colleagues. "Wow, Bill, you really nailed that diagnosis, congratulations." Second, the doctor knows that his diagnosis contains some element of guesswork. He wants the assurance that he was correct as much as the patient does. Third, the competent and caring doctor cares enough about you, his patient, to want to get this thing right. Finally, the doctor knows that it is always possible for things to turn out badly. So, somewhat selfishly, he want the patient to know that there was a second or even a third opinion to provide the best possible basis for going ahead.

If you ask your doctor for a second opinion and he hesitates for even a nanosecond to agree, you are dealing

The Second Opinion: Don't Proceed Without It

with a doctor you do not want. Either he is afraid that the second opinion will show him up for being incompetent, he has such a big ego he can't believe that he could be wrong, or he doesn't care enough about you to make sure to get it right. In any case, inform him that you are leaving and that you are going to seek another doctor.

It may be that your insurance will not pay for second opinion. That is, of course, another of the problems with the American medical system. But then it is up to you, as a Professional Patient, to decide what a second opinion is worth. Given everything we have said above, though, I hope you will move ahead and get the assurance that a second opinion can provide.

Rush to Judgment

When I was working on the cardiac floor, the following was a common scenario:

My patient was admitted to the hospital last night having experienced chest pain. He has received a cardiology work-up, and now the cardiologist comes into his room.

Cardiologist: "Don, I've looked at the results of the scan we made of your heart. You have three pretty significant partial blockages in your coronary arteries." At this point, the doctor holds up a "map" of the patient's heart. He points out the specific areas in which blockages were detected. He says, "Don, I think that you're a candidate for open heart surgery. I'll arrange for the surgeon to come and talk to you about it."

Shortly thereafter the cardiac surgeon enters the patient's room and says, "Don, I've talked to your cardiologist. He showed me the results of the tests you had at last night, and I agree that you are a candidate for open heart surgery." At this point, the surgeon shows the patient the same "map" as was shown by the cardiologist. He points out there are blockages and then informs the patient that there is a 5 percent risk of death in this surgery but that, given the seriousness of the problem, the surgery needs to be done.

At this point the surgeon asks the patient if he has any questions. The patient has only just found out that he has a problem. He has no idea of what questions he needs to ask. And so, far too often, the patient remains silent. The surgeon then turns to me, the nurse, and tells me to get the consent for surgery signed—the surgery will be scheduled for tomorrow morning.

Conclusion: The second opinion should be a standard component of medical decision-making. The costs are too great and the dangers too real not to follow this path. One final value of the second opinion needs to be mentioned. Every medical procedure, particularly surgery, has to involve some degree of anxiety on the part of the patient. To the

The Second Opinion: Don't Proceed Without It

degree that a second opinion provides any greater degree of confidence in the doctor and the procedure, this, too, is an advantage to the patient.

notes:

_____

_____

_____

_____

_____

_____

_____

_____

_____

_____

_____

_____

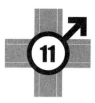

A Checklist for the Professional Patient

A Caution

The following list is not meant to be inclusive of all the knowledge and skills required for you to be a Professional Patient. It is meant, rather, to guide you to further investigation and learning as you continue to maintain and improve your health. If, because of sickness or injury, you must become an inpatient, it is meant as a guide to allow you to receive maximum benefit and to avoid the inherent dangers you will face.

- The Professional Patient has researched his family medical history. He knows as much as possible about the medical history of parents, uncles and aunts, cousins, siblings, and his own. He critically looks at his lifestyle and seeks to maximize its health-promoting aspects while reducing those that endanger health and wellness.

- The Professional Patient has a primary care doctor with whom he has a partnership based on mutual trust and confidence.

- The Professional Patient carries with him at all times a record of his medical history and current condition.

To do this, go to www.medids.com. Scroll down to the Medical I.D. Card. Fill in the information requested, print the card. Make sure that when there is any change in your status or the medications listed on the card that you print a new card. Worse than giving no information to medical personnel is giving wrong information because then they think they know what they are doing. If the Professional Patient has a complex medical history with many specialty doctors and many locations, it is a good idea to have all the medical records available.

- The Professional Patient has enacted a Durable Power of Attorney for Health Care (DPO).

In most states, the legal forms necessary to enact the DPOAHC can be found by entering "Durable Power of Attorney for Health Care" followed by the name of your state on your search engine. In some cases there may be a fee. If forms are not available online, see your attorney.

- The Professional Patient has enacted a Living Will.

- The Professional Patient follows his doctor's plan for early testing and diagnosis.

- The Professional Patient understands the dangers inherent in any hospitalization and takes all appropriate steps to maximize safety. (See Chapter 6.)

- The Professional Patient uses available library and Internet resources to became as fully informed as possible about the latest science of health and wellness. He critically evaluates all sources of medical information to weed out those that are wrong or even fraudulent.

notes:

_____

_____

_____

_____

_____

_____

_____

_____

A Checklist for the Professional Patient

Critical Questions, Tough Decisions

Throughout history, the end of life has been something beyond human control. Except in the case of suicide, death was something that simply happened. There was little or no thought of conducting a "courageous battle" against death, if only because there were no weapons with which to wage such a battle. We have now, however, come into a new time, a time in which death has become subject to human control, at least as to its time if not completely as to its manner. What is lacking and only slowly emerging is an understanding of the process of dying and an ethic to guide decisions about death.

Perhaps the most significant consequence of the development of medical technology over the last 60 years has been the extension of life expectancy in the United States from 54 to nearly 80. For millions of people, the end of life has become a process rather than an event. Sixty years ago there were no hospices in the United States. There was no need for hospice care because death, when it came, generally came quickly. Measles, mumps, scarlet fever, diphtheria, polio, smallpox, and dozens of other diseases took life—and most often took it quickly. There was little, if anything, the doctor could do. Through all of history and for the first half of the 20th century, dying was easy.

From its inception, the primary purpose of medical science, in all of its forms, was to cure illness and to repair trauma. And throughout almost all of its history, medical science, in all of its forms, was largely incapable of doing much to accomplish either goal. Then, beginning in the middle of the 20th century, the practice of medicine began to develop the skills that allowed it to cure diseases that had, for centuries, led to almost certain death and to repair injuries that, for centuries, produced permanent incapacitation and, far too often, death.

Sixty years ago the odds were that if a person needed a doctor, the doctor came to the house. At that time, the doctor could carry almost every medical instrument and every available medication in the famous "black bag." Prior to the development of large hospitals, babies were born at home, medical care was given at home, and death occurred at home. Death was, if not welcome, at least familiar. Then the institution of the hospital changed everything. The hospital became the place for coming into life, and for leaving it. The baby came into the world, unobserved by anybody but the doctor and the attending nurses. The notion of having the father or members of a family present at the delivery simply disappeared.

A similar development has occurred with respect to dying. The goal of medicine is now to deny death for as long as possible. This requires that the dying person be treated for whatever it is that is causing the death. The treatment normally occurs in the hospital as, of course, does the dying. The treatment and the dying most often occur in isolation from family or friends. Until quite recently children were not

Look but Don't Touch

Our daughter Elizabeth is 43 years old. Just two years before she was born, my wife, Rosalie, along with another woman, began to teach the Lamaze method for birthing in Green Bay. A core element of this method is to have the father or some other member of the family or a friend "coach" the mother through the delivery. Although today the Lamaze and similar methods have come into the medical mainstream, just 40 years ago they were foreign to the practice of medicine. Mothers trained in the method may have been allowed to have their coach with them through the process of labor, but when it came time for the delivery, they were alone. I coached Rosalie through hours of labor and then watched her wheeled into the delivery room while I waited outside. After a period of time, Elizabeth was brought to me, wrapped in a blanket. I was given a quick look and then she was returned to the nursery. I was not allowed to hold her for a week.

Critical Questions, Tough Decisions

allowed to leave the lobby of the hospital to visit the patient. It is common for family and friends to be asked to leave the room whenever medical care is being delivered. Thus, very few people ever experience either the miracle of birth or the moment of death. The experience of death has become that of viewing the fully clothed and highly cosmeticized corpse lying in a velvet-lined casket. Rather than being a familiar and accepted part of life, death has become something strange, fearful, and to be deferred or avoided at all costs.

High-Risk Babies, Then and Now

Our daughter, Elizabeth, was born on Christmas Day, 1967. I was 32 years old and a college professor. Rosalie was a librarian and 30 years old. The belief at that time was that women should not bear children when they were 30 years old or older because of the increased incidence of birth defects such as a Down syndrome.

I went to see Rosalie's ob-gyn. I asked him what the protocols were if our child should be born with significant defects. He seemed quite disturbed at my request, as if my asking might somehow jinx the outcome. He explained to me that when babies were born who clearly had defects that could be life threatening or that might threaten a good quality of life, the protocol was to place the infant in an isolette, set it aside, and wait 24 hours. If, at the end of that time, the baby was still alive, then everything possible would be done to keep it alive.

Whatever the condition of the infant 40 years ago, there was little that the doctor could have done anyway. Today, though, that situation has changed dramatically. While in nursing school, I took a course in infant and child development. A nurse from the high-risk neonatal intensive care unit (NICU) of a local hospital came to speak to the class. She explained to us with evident pride that we now had the technological capacity to "save" babies with birth weights as low as a pound and a half and maybe even lower. She displayed for us a cap for these infants that was made by a volunteer who did this kind of thing. The model on which the cap was knitted was the rind of half an orange.

I came away from that experience with the realization that the very low birth weight infant is looked upon by the medical profession as a challenge. The challenge is to make certain that the infant does not die. Anything and everything possible will be done to ensure this outcome.

The point is this: when Elizabeth was born, there was virtually nothing that could be done to keep her alive if her birth was accompanied by extremely low birth weight or many other life-threatening kinds of defects. Today, on the contrary, very low birth weight infants will be kept alive. They

Critical Questions, Tough Decisions

will in all probability (and the scientific evidence is quite clear on this point) experience lifelong problems. Chief among these are mental retardation, cerebral palsy, and chronic cardiac and respiratory problems. Once again, then, we are confronted with another new ethical issue. What is the obligation of parents or of society to use medical technology for the sake of "saving" extremely low birth weight babies? Must we continue to "do everything?" If the answer to that question is negative, what then are the criteria to be used in determining when the baby should be allowed to die?

Paralleling the development of powerful medical technology came the creation of private medical insurance (inappropriately called "health insurance") and, in the 1960s, the creation of Medicare for the elderly and Medicaid for the poor. Suddenly the cost of medical care became a matter of relative indifference to the patient and the patient's family as long as they had insurance, either private or from the government. For those without such insurance, however, the cost of medical care could lead to bankruptcy. Life was lived in the constant fear of a medical need that could send the family into the streets to beg.

All of these things—the creation of the modern hospital, the development of "miracle" drugs and medications, the creation of sophisticated surgical procedures, the isolation of family from the experiences of birth and death, and the divorce of the patient from the financial costs of medicine[1] have led us to our current situation.

Ethical Questions Unanswered

Still Comatose

My patient was a 72-year-old farmer, 72 hours out of open heart surgery. During the surgery, he had had a stroke, a massive stroke. He was comatose. A neurological consult that had been ordered, and I was asked to assist. Following a thorough examination, the neurologist went to the nursing station and made a note in the patient's chart. He stated that the patient had had a serious stroke and that rehabilitation was not a reasonable possibility. He recommended that all hydration be terminated and that the patient be allowed to die. Shortly thereafter, the patient's cardiologist came to the floor. He read the chart and went into the patient's room to meet with the family. Thirty minutes later he returned to the nursing station, read the neurologist's note in the patient chart, and wrote an order in the chart to start an IV of D5 W (a solution that would keep the patient hydrated). When I asked him why we were doing this, his response was that it was what the family wanted. The patient subsequently recovered from his open heart surgery and was discharged, still comatose, to a nursing home.

---

1   Given the quickening pace at which families are losing health insurance and thereby facing the potentially devastating costs of medical care, the issue of when to terminate medical care for people who are elderly or very sick will need to be confronted. If insurance companies are allowed to refuse coverage to people because of pre-existing conditions, might families who lack medical insurance be allowed to stop payment for the care of a family member for whose care the costs have become ruinous to the point of bankruptcy? And at that point, the question arises as to the responsibility of society to continue to pay the costs of ongoing care.

Critical Questions, Tough Decisions

The point here is that the family had no immediate liability for the cost of care associated with their request that "everything be done." Like many, they felt that the failure to "do everything" would be tantamount to killing the patient. It may also have been that they held the belief that holding on long enough might open the doors to the possibility that a new cure or treatment would be found. And so in the face of hope that things could turn out okay and not facing any immediate financial liability for the costs of continuing care, this family and thousands even millions of others press the medical system to "do everything."

And elements of the medical system, driven to maximize revenue, are often only too happy to agree. On the other side of this coin is the practice of some hospitals to actually discharge indigent patients into the streets from for-profit hospitals and some private and not-for-profit hospitals to publicly owned facilities. This practice, commonly called, "dumping," has been documented across the country, and in some states laws have been enacted to stop it.

There is an irony in the fact that for the 40 million uninsured Americans and even for those with insurance, the costs of medical care have become prohibitive for families as well as for society. And this occurs just at the time that people feel the obligation to insist that "everything be done." Medical benefits, even those provided in the best of insurance policies, can be exhausted, and when the benefits have been used up, families are required to assume the burdens of paying for medical care themselves. They are then torn between the between the felt obligation to do everything possible and the recognition that the consequence of fulfilling his obligation can be and often is bankruptcy.

Families are forced into bankruptcy in their efforts to provide for the care of elderly parents. Children are forced to forego fulfilling their own retirement dreams as their lives are invested in caring for an elderly parent or relative. The larger society is forced to defer the realization of many of its goals: the improvement of education, the maintenance of the country's infrastructure, the development of arts and culture, and the protection of the environment, as well as many other desired and desirable outcomes as the demands of medical care, invested merely in deferring death, dominate public understanding, law, and ethics.

Millions of people live in nursing homes, being kept alive with medications and surgeries even though they are no longer able to provide even the most basic self-cares and even though, it can be reasonably judged, they have no quality of life. Often they are kept alive even though they may, with full understanding, knowingly and repeatedly request that they be allowed to die.[2]

The negative impacts of the uncritical application of medical science to the maintenance of life have become clearer to growing numbers of people. These people have to confront the sometimes unbearable costs of medical care and the deferral of their own life dreams because of the demands of caring for family members no longer capable of caring for themselves.

At the same time as there is a growing awareness of and commitment to the demands of health and wellness throughout the United States, there is the parallel, largely inarticulate, growing awareness of the need—and even the responsibility—to treat death and dying as processes that are now subject, as they never have been before in history, to decision. Medical science has developed the capacity to prolong life almost indefinitely. Tragically, there has not been a parallel development of an ethic to guide the process for deciding when it is time to walk away from medicine and allow death to occur. As individuals, as families, and as a society, it becomes more important every day to come to an understanding of this issue.

---

2   There may be a kind of catch-22 involved in this. It might be argued that a person should be allowed to die when they are no longer mentally competent. However, if a person is mentally competent enough to request their own death, they cannot be allowed to die.

Some Food for Thought

I cannot hope within this context to offer more than a partial examination of the questions and issues involved in developing an ethic for the end of life. Following, though, is at the least the beginning of such an examination.

Consider the case of my mother-in-law, Camille. She was wife to her husband, Earl. She was a mother to six children, five girls and a boy. She was in every respect a wonderful person. In her mid-80s, though, she began to experience episodes of forgetfulness. With increasing frequency, she would become faint and often fall. Following the death of Earl, she moved in with a daughter and her husband who lived close by. They loved her and she loved them, and for years they were happy together. Yet as her episodes of forgetfulness became a kind of dementia and she began to experience more and more falls, it became difficult and even dangerous for her daughter and son-in-law to provide her daily care. Reluctantly they moved her into a nearby nursing home.

Only a matter of weeks after she entered the nursing home it was Christmas. The family, including the five remaining children, gathered. The first thing to do was to visit Camille. She was unable to recognize or name any of her children. The happy, laughing, and delightful person that

Critical Questions, Tough Decisions

she had been all of her life was gone. A conversation with her doctor revealed that she was being given three medications whose purpose was to keep her heart beating, to control its rhythm, and to keep her kidneys working. Following a family discussion, it was decided to request that the doctor remove the orders for those three medications and to take only those steps necessary to keep Camille free from pain.

The medications were discontinued. Three days later Camille died peacefully in her sleep.

What is to be thought of this tale? Many, if not most, of those to whom this story has been related agree strongly that the family had made an appropriate decision. They agree that the doctor responded correctly. At the same time, there are strong voices, both individual and institutional, that would argue that it was wrong for the doctor to withhold life-preserving medical treatment and for the family to have requested it.

This and similar disagreements dealing with issues from contraception to abortion to the use of "heroic"[3] measures

---

3   As medical technology has made it possible to prolong respiration and heartbeat (historically the two necessary signs of life) almost indefinitely, leading figures in theology and medical ethics have come to the conclusion that there is no obligation to provide "extraordinary" or "heroic "measures to prolong a person's life. The immediate and continuing question has to do with how to define a medical intervention as either extraordinary or heroic. Rather than solving the problem of deciding when and under what circumstances to end medical treatment, the concepts of extraordinary and heroic care have simply shifted the terms of the discussion. This has not solved the problem.

to prolong life—and ending with the maintenance of people who are old and incurably sick—tear at the fabric of American society. These are not disagreements that one can choose not to be involved in, for that very choice constitutes a choice to retain the status quo, whatever that might be.

The presidential election of 2008 found the issue of abortion to be one of the most significant questions facing Democratic and Republican parties and the electorate. At issue was the likelihood that the winning party would have the opportunity to replace two justices on the Supreme Court, two justices, who, depending on their approach to the abortion question, could overturn Roe vs. Wade, the 1972 decision that made abortion a legal alternative for a woman in the United States. Such a decision would be at least as divisive as and probably more divisive to American society than the original decision.

The notoriety achieved by the career of Dr. Jack Kevorkian, with his commitment to assisting his patients to end their own lives, in some cases with his direct assistance, is further evidence of the divisiveness created by the end-of-life issue.

Further evidence of the degree of social controversy regarding the determination of the end-of-life is illustraated by the case of Terri Schiavo, as mentioned in an earlier chapter. Here it took the combined efforts of the office of the president, of Congress, and of the Supreme Court to arrive at what was at best a highly controversial ruling that a feeding tube could be removed from the body of a woman adjudged to have been in a persistent vegetative state for 15 years.

The case of Camille, then, is like millions of similar cases. Now that we have the ability to maintain heartbeat and respiration for an almost indefinite period of time, the issue becomes when and how should the decision to be made to allow death to occur? The answer to this question will be a long time in coming. Yet given society's ambivalence regarding what the right answer is, there are things that each person and family can do, each in the light of their own beliefs, to facilitate a response that they believe is appropriate.

First and most important is to talk about the issue. Perhaps nothing is more difficult to confront and to discuss than death. Yet it is increasingly important that we do just that. Death will happen. Again, either we, each of us, take charge of determining when and under what circumstances it will occur, or we make ourselves hostages to the medical system. We are the CEOs of our lives, like it or not. So it's time for family discussion, for creating a living will, for having a Durable Power of Attorney for Health Care, and for considering programs like hospice and palliative care.

notes:

_____

_____

_____

_____

_____

_____

_____

_____

_____

_____

_____

_____

_____

_____

_____

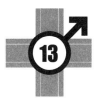

Advanced Directives and Other Matters

As has been said so many times before in this book, modern medicine has made it possible to prolong life almost indefinitely. A consequence of this fact is that the time and manner of death have now become, as never before in all of history, a matter of choice. We will die, that's a given. How and when we will die is now to a very large degree up to us. The Professional Patient packs in his medical tool kit the instruments we will now discuss. Through their wise use he takes control of what may be, besides birth, the most important event of all. Three of these tools are called "Advanced Directives." The other tools are available as the end of life approaches and provide control over the matters of pain and suffering.

Advanced Directives

Through advanced directives, patients give directions as to the kind and amount of medical care that they want when they are not capable of directly expressing their wishes. In particular, the advanced directive normally describes the kind of care that should be given in case of an illness from which recovery is unlikely. Advanced directives can be used by patients who have a chronic condition that may not cause immediate death but that is being controlled through the use of procedures, e.g. intubation for breathing or use of a feeding tube which, in the mind of the patient, are so onerous that they should not be used or continued. Advance directives usually tell the doctor what kinds of treatment are not to be given. They may also give directions as to desired kinds or levels of care.

There are three kinds of advanced directive: the durable power of attorney for health care, the living will, and the "do not resuscitate" order.

The Durable Power of Attorney for Health Care

The first and most important advanced directive for anyone to make is the durable power of attorney for health (medical) care. The durable power of attorney (DPOA) is the vehicle through which an individual gives another person the legal authority to act on her behalf at the point at which she is no longer capable of providing direction herself.

The durable power of attorney can be enacted in almost

every state without the requirement that an attorney be involved. Access to the legal documents required to establish a durable power of attorney is available on the Internet for most states. In that document, the individual specifies who they desire to have the power, the conditions under which they desire to have the power enacted, and the decisions available to the person designated. [1]

It is important that every member of the patient's family understand and agree to the terms of the DPOA. Given the tendency and incentives for the medical system to continue treatment, regardless of reasonably anticipated outcomes, it often happens that a relative may suddenly appear on the scene and order that those conditions be set aside. In such situations, representatives of the medical system will often defer to the dissenting opinion.

The Living Will

A second important component for end-of-life decisions is the living will. Most often this document can be included in the durable power of attorney for health care. Coming to the end of life without a living will can jeopardize not

---

1   Using Google or almost any other browser, simply enter "Durable Power of Attorney for Health Care" followed by the name of a state. The necessary documents can be downloaded. In some cases, there may be a minimal charge for the download. Once downloaded, the documents provide instructions as to how they are to be completed. They should be signed by the person to whom the DPOA is being assigned and then notarized. When the patient enters the medical system, he or she will usually be asked to provide a copy of the DPOA

Advanced Directives and Other Matters

only the patient but the patient's family. The living will sets forward the conditions under which the patient desires to have life-sustaining treatments continued or terminated. The primary care doctor should almost always be involved in the preparation of a living will. The doctor's expertise in the kinds of matters with which the living will deals and the doctor's knowledge of the patient and the patient's family (in the best of all possible worlds) can be invaluable in preparing a document that fully and accurately expresses the informed desires of the patient.

Again, everyone in the patient's family should be informed of the contents of the living will to avoid any last minute complications if there should be someone who decides to object.

The Do Not Resuscitate Order

Of special importance is the "do not resuscitate" (DNR) advanced directive. The DNR order comes into play when the heart stops beating or breathing stops. The do not resuscitate order says that when the heart should cease or breathing should stop, no efforts will be made to restore either. Without that order in effect, representatives of the medical system, emergency medical technicians, emergency room personnel, hospital staff, and the staff in nursing homes and other long-term care facilities have no choice but

That Guy Nurse

to bring every possible effort to bear to restore heartbeat and respirations regardless of the conditions leading to the heart failure or the likely outcomes of restoring a heartbeat.

Once a patient has determined that he wants to be a "no code" (not to be resuscitated if his heart should stop), it is important that all family members be notified and that they agree that they will not act to intervene if the patient's heart stops or breathing ceases.

If the patient is in a hospital or nursing home, those facilities must be notified of the patient's DNR status and by law they must abide by it. If the patient is in home care, the DNR status must be prominently displayed (often with a bracelet). Otherwise, if an emergency medical team should be called to the home and heartbeat or respiration should stop, they must, by law, take every possible measure to restore the patient.

The decision to choose DNR status must be done in consultation with the primary care doctor. The DPOA should also include the DNR order.

Hospice Care

Consider how you will feel as you approach the end of your life. If you are like the great majority of people, you will not fear actually dying as much as you fear the pain and

Advanced Directives and Other Matters

suffering that we associate with that time. We understand when we stop to ponder that we will die. We don't want it too soon, but we know that it will happen sometime. What frightens us, what we worry about, is that we will experience pain, lots of pain, for a long time. Sadly, that is often the case. Yet it need not be.

The ability to control pain is one of the great advances of modern medicine. Unfortunately, pain is almost always a moving target. Managing pain requires the ability to make ever-changing responses in terms of the medications used, their dosage, and even the choice to use non-pharmaceutical means, such as heat or cold, pressure or relief from pressure, massage, or any of the other techniques that have proven to be effective depending on the kind, cause, and location of the pain. The point is that dealing with pain requires constant attention and the availability of the means to relieve or eliminate the problem.

Further complicating the problem of pain and management is the fact that many patients, probably most, prefer dealing with a moderate level of pain versus receiving the kind of pain relief that leaves them essentially unconscious. What it boils down to is this: pain control requires an ongoing dialogue between the patient, or the patient's advocate, and the doctor or nurse who have the ability to decide what needs to be done.

This brings us to hospice. The creation of the hospice is another of the products of modern medicine. Only a few decades ago, there were no hospices in the United States. Why? Because dying normally happened rather quickly and because there was little medical knowledge of pain or of how it could be controlled, which is one of the primary tasks of hospice. The focus of medicine was on curing sickness, repairing trauma, and prolonging life, but the medical establishment was not very good at accomplishing any of these things. It was only in the 1950s that this situation began to change and to change dramatically.

With those changes came the ability to prolong life, and with that ability came the need to deal with pain that could be not only severe but that could last for weeks, months, and even years. As the pharmaceutical industry created more and more new medications and as surgeries became ever more complex, there was a parallel development of the field of pain control.

Dying, whether from cancer or heart disease or diabetes or any of a number of other causes, began to take longer and longer to accomplish, and the modern hospice organization came into being. The role of the hospice is to support both the patient and the patient's family when it has been determined that death is most likely only a matter of a few months away and that nothing can be done medically to

Advanced Directives and Other Matters

change that outcome. The hospice team, consisting of a doctor, a nurse, a social worker, and often a clergyperson, are constantly available to the patient and to the family to respond to the issues of pain and grief and all of the other problems and concerns that can arise.

A Common Hospice Experience

Tuesday afternoon. My hospice social work partner and I head out of town to a rural nursing home to do an admission assessment. We arrive and find that our patient is already in the process of active dying. She is unresponsive. Her legs are mottled. Her forehead is burning with fever, and her hands and feet are icy cold. We hear the death rattles in her lungs, which have filled with fluid.

We proceed to do our assessment and fill in the necessary paperwork to accomplish admission to hospice. All the while we are doing this, we glance at each other and shake our heads over the thought that had we been called weeks or even months before, so much suffering for both our patient and for her family could have been averted. However, the family had kept holding out hope that this situation might improve. It was only when it was completely clear that death was close was hospice called.

We finished our work, packed up, and headed back to the car. A voice called, "Nurse, come back." We returned. Our patient was dead. I then did the last work of hospice. I prepared the body to be delivered to the funeral home. I called her doctor to pronounce the death. I called the coroner. I inventoried her medications to return them to hospice for disposal. I gave what consolation I could to her family. We left.

That Guy Nurse

In my opinion, the greatest value of hospice lies in its ability to respond quickly and effectively to pain. Because of this, and because pain management requires constant attention, hospice is a blessing to the millions of patients and families who have become part of the hospice movement. Do not be afraid to seek the assistance of your local hospice. One of the saddest facts about the American medical system is that the average stay in hospice is less than four weeks, and not uncommonly it is only a matter of days or even hours.

Early in my career as a hospice nurse, I realized that many of the families with whom I was working had waited until the doctor suggested that it would be appropriate for the patient to enter hospice. The doctor, however, has a number of reasons not to make a hospice referral. First, doctors are often afraid that if they suggest that a hospice referral is appropriate, the patient's family will become angry and announce that they're going to find another doctor, one who will not "give up". Second, there are doctors who are themselves not willing to give up on the patient. In all sincerity, they believe that if death can be deferred for any length of time, a cure may be found or a surgical intervention created that could return the patient to health. It is not within their belief system to refer patients to hospice because the referral accepts the fact that nothing more will be done to attempt to cure whatever it is that has brought the patient to their

Advanced Directives and Other Matters

current situation.

It must be understood that entering hospice is not a matter of giving up. Rather, the decision to enter hospice is the recognition that life does come to an end regardless of how much medicine may try to overcome that fact. It is the recognition that death is approaching and that the best thing for the patient and for those who love him is to do everything possible to make the passage as free from pain and suffering as possible.

If ever a patient or family think that it might be appropriate to seek hospice care, they need only to call a local hospice and request an evaluation. The hospice will respond by sending a nurse and a social worker to do an evaluation. If, in their opinion, hospice care would be appropriate, they will contact the doctor. Almost always the doctor, relieved to have the decision taken out of his hands, will agree and make the referral.

Palliative Care

Corresponding with but expanding the idea of hospice care is the growth of a new medical specialty in palliative care. Palliative care is designed to provide symptom control for patients whose quality of life is significantly altered by reason of an injury or disease that is not terminal in the sense of having a prognosis of six months of life or less. Palliative care recognizes that, even while there are ongoing efforts to cure a condition, the symptoms associated with that condition may be harmful to good quality of life. Thus, the commitment of palliative care is to relieve or to manage the suffering of both patient and family related to symptoms such as pain, difficulty breathing, fatigue, loss of appetite, nausea, and stress.

Although a symptom relief is a primary goal of hospice care, there are ongoing problems with the management and relief of symptoms and other areas of the medical system. Time, energy, and money are often spent to achieve cure while symptom management simply takes a back seat. Pain relief itself is an emerging medical specialty. Unfortunately, too often it takes a back seat to the focus on cure. The Professional Patient is aware that unless the symptoms of disease or injury are relieved, the efforts at cure will themselves be rendered less effective. The Professional Patient therefore requests and pursues palliative care whenever symptoms begin to affect the patient's quality of life.

Advanced Directives and Other Matters

notes:

_____

_____

_____

_____

_____

_____

_____

_____

_____

_____

_____

_____

_____

_____

Notes From ThatGuyNurse arises from and points to a vision for the future of medical care in the United States of America. Achieving this vision will entail changes in every area of medical practice: governmental (the role and function of the government), private (the roles of private insurance and of employers), practice (roles of primary care doctors, of specialists, and of adjunct personnel such as nurses, nurse practitioners, and physician's assistants), and—this is perhaps the most important part of the vision—the new roles to be played by the patient.

A Note on the Purpose of a "Vision"

A term "vision," as used here, is a picture of an ideal state of affairs. It is a picture of what the American medical system could be and should be if it is to become a genuine health care system. The purpose of the vision is to give inspiration and direction to everyone who is involved with and affected by the system. *I hope it will energize you, the reader, to become involved not just in your own health but also in your role as a citizen to work for its achievement.*

It is not an objection to this vision to point out that it is impractical and that it will be exceedingly difficult to achieve.

251

Part IV: A Vision for the Future of Medial Practice in the U.S.

In fact, if it were practical and easily achieved, it would not be a vision. It would be a plan. This vision will, if enough people adopt it, become the basis of a plan, a plan to remake the American medical system. My intention is that this vision will be inspiring, clear, and challenging to all who read it.

The Vision

The vision consists of seven parts, or scenes, each speaking to one dimension of the way in which health care is practiced in the United States today. Together these parts form a comprehensive picture of what can be.

Before embarking on the task of describing this vision, I want to be clear about a point that is subject to considerable controversy. The question is whether people have a right to medical care. I believe that access to basic medical care should be regarded as a right in the United States. I find it ethically objectionable that people are forced to beg for medical care, particularly when innocent persons suffer or die for the lack of that care. I find it ethically objectionable that millions are forced to live in the constant dread of needing medical attention without access to medical insurance because of pre-existing conditions. I find it ethically objectionable that the leading cause of bankruptcy in the United States is the inability of individuals and families to pay the costs of medical care. This list could go on, but I think the point has been made.

It is important to understand what it means to say that someone has a "right" to medical care. It means that, all other conditions being equal, society has an obligation to provide that care. In the statement of a vision for the future of medical care below, it will be made clear that there are conditions that take away the right. That is, it is not an unconditional right.

The seven parts are these:

1. Primary care medicine will be established as the foundation of the American medical system.

2. Patients will be responsible for paying for primary care services, on a sliding fee scale based on ability to pay.

3. For medical procedures exceeding a reasonable charge to the patient (based upon patient ability to pay), there will be a single-payer mechanism operated by or overseen by government.

4. Primary care physicians will be compensated, in addition to the compensation provided by patients, on a scale that recognizes their contributions to prevention and the long-term health and wellness of their patients.

Part IV: A Vision for the Future of Medial Practice in the U.S.

5. Care for chronic medical conditions whose causes lie outside the control of patients (for example, Type 1 diabetes) will be provided by the single payer, again with the understanding that the patient will be financially responsible for that care to the extent determined by the patient's ability to pay.

6. Employers will be released from any obligation to pay the costs of medical care for their employees or employees' families.

7. Decisions to forsake treatment aimed at cure and to initiate palliative care will be make by physician panels with patients and families having the opportunity, should they disagree with a panel decision, to both appeal and/or to assume the costs of care.

1. Primary care medicine will be established as the foundation of the American medical system.

- The primary care doctor will be placed at the center of medical care through a system that allows the primary care doctor and his patients to develop long-term relationships.

- Preventive care and teaching will become the focus

That Guy Nurse

and emphasis of primary care medicine.

- All proposed changes in the medical system will be judged by their effect on the practice of primary care medicine and on the patient/physician relationship.

Most current public discussion on problems with the American medical system is focused on the issue of costs. Relatively little attention is given to the kind of medical care being offered. Almost ignored is the fact that the bulk of the money being spent for medical care is being spent for the treatment of preventable conditions.

Two conditions define what it is to be a preventable medical condition. The first involves the patient understanding and then acting in such ways as to reduce or eliminate the conditions and behaviors that contribute to, and may even cause, the condition in question. For example, obesity, smoking, failure to exercise, and unmanaged stress contribute to or cause those disease states that, today, lead to nearly 50 percent of deaths in the United States. These are all preventable conditions. Some experts claim that up to 70 percent of medical costs are for the treatment of conditions that are, in principle, preventable.

The obvious vehicle for preventive care is the primary care physician. Yet it is precisely at the level of primary care that system managers, both governmental and the managers

Part IV: A Vision for the Future of Medial Practice in the U.S.

of private insurance, seek to achieve savings by requiring that primary care doctors spend an average of only six to 10 minutes with each patient per visit. And this is primary care for which patients are expected to pay first-dollars out of pocket while the much more expensive specialty care is covered by employer-provided insurance. In the area of primary care, the role of the doctor is being taken over by nurse practitioners and physician's assistants who, because of the growing emphasis on cost, are available much more cheaply than are medical doctors.

Yet in the face of a growing need for primary care physicians, the supply of these doctors is either frozen or dropping as students entering medical school opt for the more prestigious and high-income specialty programs. For the past 20 years or more, the compensation provided to primary care doctors has been declining. The primary care doctor is now at the bottom and of the medical pecking order. Social status is conferred on the specialists, the cardiologists and gastroenterologists and orthopedic surgeons.[1]

---

1   In a study recently published in the *Archives of Internal Medicine*, med students surveyed in 1990 and 2007 about their attitudes toward internal medicine careers. According to the *Wall Street Journal*, the study "finds that while about the same percentage of med students–23 percent in the earlier survey of 1,244 students, and 24 percent in the later survey of 1,177 students–plan internal medicine careers, the proportion planning to go into primary care fell to 2 percent from 9 percent." Additionally, "the appeal of primary care as a reason to go into internal medicine fell to 33 percent from 57 percent."
As the healthcare landscape has shifted in recent years, the appeal of primary care has, too. Lower pay, longer hours, more patients, limited Medicare reimbursements, and little interaction with patients is reason enough to go into specialty medicine.

That Guy Nurse

The primary care doctor can and must be the foundation of anything that dares to call itself a health care system. The primary care doctor is not just the point of entry into the medical system, she is the person whose knowledge and skill can eliminate up to 70 percent of the costs of medical care in the United States and who can, at the same time, eliminate up to 70 percent of the pain and suffering and disability that are the reasons for all of that spending.

If a patient and a doctor are to have a fruitful relationship, there must be trust. In order to be effective, the doctor must have the broadest possible base of knowledge about the patient, the patient's history, the patient's life, the patient's values, and the hopes and fears that guide the patient's choices as well as the most intimate facets of the patient's daily life. All of these things and more contribute to the task of diagnosis and to the development of effective plans of care. Yet today primary care medicine is practiced on a model that requires physicians to see 25 or more patients every day, to spend an average of only six to 10 minutes with each patient for each visit, and to build and maintain a panel of not less than 3,000 patients. The current practice of primary medicine could not be more antithetical to the fundamental requirements of good and effective medical practice. Trust can only be built on experience, long-term experience, during which the physician learns to trust the patient and

Part IV: A Vision for the Future of Medial Practice in the U.S.

the patient's description of symptoms and concerns and during which the patient comes to trust the doctor's skill and knowledge.

The current practice of medicine makes it almost impossible to maintain a long-term relationship between a patient and a doctor. If the patient's employer chooses to move to a different insurance company, it is common that the patient is required to find a new doctor at a new clinic. Even when a patient retains the same primary care doctor, often when the patient needs to see the doctor, the doctor is simply not available and the patient sees whichever doctor is on call. Hospitalization today almost requires that a patient see and deal with a physician other than his primary care doctor. We have created a new class of physicians called "hospitalists" whose job is to see the patients that other doctors send to the hospital. What at one time was the rule—patient and the doctor working together over a period of years and even a lifetime—has now become the exception.

This vision holds forth a future in which the doctor/patient relationship looks much the same as it did in the middle of the last century. Doctors will have fewer patients and will be able to spend the time necessary to learn about their patients. Patients will have the opportunity to know their doctors. Doctors will be able to work with patients for as long as that relationship is fruitful and mutually satisfactory.

Doctors will be able to accompany their patients when it is necessary to visit a specialist and thereby to ensure that the patient's questions are answered and that the answers are understood. Doctors might even be able, if circumstances warrant, to go to a patient's home to provide care, while the patient remains not just in the comfort but in the security of that place.

The question is often raised as to how this could possibly ever happen with anything like the current number of practicing primary care physicians. The answer lies in the conviction that when patients have knowledge of how to maintain their health and when they practice prevention and when they know when and where to enter the medical system, there will be enough physicians. [2]

I have met and worked with many physicians who have become embittered and skeptical about the idea that patients can and will learn to be effective self-advocates for health and wellness. Although they began the practice of medicine with the ideal of working in partnership with their patients with a mutual goal of achieving and maintaining health,

---

2   A mark of how unbalanced current medical practice has become is the fact that the number of medical students seeking careers in primary care medicine is shrinking rapidly as more and more students choose specialty practice both for its prestige and its greatly enhanced income potential. On February 12, 2008, the Governmental Accountability Office report to Congress on supply trends for primary care physicians stated that by 2020, the country will be 65,950 doctors short of what will be needed. This presupposes that the practice of primary medicine will not substantially change and that doctors will still be seeing 20 to 25 patients per day.

Part IV: A Vision for the Future of Medial Practice in the U.S.

they became skeptical and embittered as they experienced hundreds and then thousands of patients who did not comply with their directions, consistently engaged in health-destructive behaviors, and then made the entrance to the doctor's office merely a revolving door for repeating and generally worsening issues that could and should have been managed at their onset.

Sisyphus was cursed by the Gods of Athens to spend all of eternity pushing a rock to the top of a mountain, only to have it immediately roll back to the bottom, where he once again had to push it to the top. The primary care physician lives a life very much like that of Sisyphus. It's no small wonder that he becomes skeptical and sometimes cynical as he faces the challenge of helping patients manage their own health and wellness. This is what happens when doctors and patients each become cogs in a massive and impersonal machine.

2. Patients will be responsible for paying for primary care services, on a sliding fee scale based on ability to pay.

Approaching the middle of the 20th century, patients and doctors stood in a primarily business relationship. The patient sought the services of the doctor and understood that there would be a charge for those services. There were no private insurance programs and no government programs to pay for medical services. What made this relationship unique was the fact that the doctor stood under a professional obligation to provide services to his patients regardless of their ability to pay.

This will not change. The doctor/patient relationship will continue with service being offered in exchange for payment.

In almost every area of life, people are held accountable for the consequences of their actions. In the arena of medicine, however, this not the case. For a variety of reasons, some historical and some psychological, this society does not generally regard behaviors that are clearly destructive of health to be matters for which individuals should be held to account. On the contrary, the more the destructive the behaviors—smoking, obesity, failure to exercise, failure to take appropriate safety precautions on motorcycles and in cars—the more it is both understood and expected that society will pay for consequences of those behaviors.

It is a deeply held belief that when a person becomes sick or injured, no matter what the reason for the sickness or injury, that person has a right to expect all the medical care that might be required to restore their condition, to the maximum degree possible, to one of health. The only condition that alters this conviction is that the person does

Part IV: A Vision for the Future of Medial Practice in the U.S.

not have medical insurance or lacks the ability to pay for their care. In that situation, assuming that the medical need is not an emergency, the patient is left to go into the streets to beg for others to provide the funds needed to pay. This is a cruel irony.

At the same time, if a person recklessly and willfully destroys their automobile or their home, there is no understanding that society has a responsibility to replace either. It seems to be different, though when we talk of sickness and injury. To suggest that a person who has been injured in an accident, even though he may have caused it himself through his own carelessness, should not receive all the available medical resources available is anathema, subject only to the condition mentioned above. This attitude lies at the base of much of what is wrong with the American medical system. There is an attitude of entitlement regarding medical care. It is an attitude that suggests that no matter what sickness or injury a person may experience, that person is entitled to all available medical care if only he has insurance or is a participant in a government program such as Medicare or Medicaid.

It must be understood that one of the fundamental reasons for the existence of the large hospital systems, of the private health insurance corporations, and of the pharmaceutical industry is to make a profit. Even hospital systems that are chartered as not-for-profit organizations behave on the whole as if their primary purpose is to make a profit. This can easily be seen by examining where, when it is time for improvements to facilities or equipment, these systems choose to invest their money. The money almost always goes to purchase the latest, high-tech surgical equipment or diagnostic machinery or to build more clinics whose purpose is to draw more patients into the system. Since these hospital systems receive little or no compensation for programs designed to promote health and wellness, they rarely invest money in such programs. Far too often proposed new programs are not evaluated in terms of their effect on the health of the community but, rather, on their potential for generating income.

In the settlement of many types of insurance claims for automobile accidents, for example, an effort is made to determine the degree of responsibility that can be attributed to the claimant, and the amount awarded to the claimant is adjusted in relation to the degree of responsibility and determined. Such determinations are never made in the case of medical insurance claims. The claimant's degree of responsibility for the condition for which medical treatment is needed is simply not considered in determining the final payment.

This vision calls for exactly this kind of calculation to be made for persons seeking to be compensated for the medical services they receive. To the degree that an individual

263

Part IV: A Vision for the Future of Medial Practice in the U.S.

may reasonably held to be responsible for having caused the sickness or injury for which they seek treatment, the compensation they receive should be adjusted.

3. For medical procedures exceeding a reasonable charge to the patient (based upon patient ability to pay), there will be a single-payer mechanism operated by or overseen by government.

Insurance coverage may be provided by private corporations that will be regulated by the government.

For example, no insurance coverage, private or governmental, will be denied because of pre-existing conditions. This may be the most controversial part of this vision. It has become virtually a self-evident truth that the United States' health care system is the best in the world and that any form of" socialized" medicine is inherently inferior. Almost everyone has heard the horror stories of people, particularly those who live in Canada, who have been unable to receive timely treatment for such immediately life-threatening conditions as cancer or heart attack. This is no more than an urban myth.

The fact is that although the United States spends far more per capita than any other developed nation in the world on medical care, it ranks only 27th in terms of longevity and

37th in terms of healthy longevity. It ranks near the bottom in infant mortality, and at the middle or below the middle in almost every measure of medical outcomes. Thirty million Americans have no access to medical insurance whatever and thereby receive no medical care until they are forced to go to a nearby emergency room, where the cost of care is immensely higher than it would have been in a primary care clinic.

Defenders of the American medical system are quick to point out that the dominant American lifestyle accounts for much of the difficulty described above. A nation that is the most obese in the world and in which people exercise less is, they point out, bound to have higher costs of medical care and poorer outcomes. Even granting this, however, the question remains as to why Americans are more obese and exercise less than most other peoples in the world. Part of the answer has to be that the American medical system is, in its current configuration, incapable of providing the information and education that people need if they are to become effective managers of their own health and wellness.

Americans have been taught that the American medical system can do miracles in providing cures for sickness and repair of trauma. They have been taught that there are myriad medicines available over the counter that can effectively remedy virtually every ailment that a person might confront,

Part IV: A Vision for the Future of Medial Practice in the U.S.

from hair loss to obesity to sexual dysfunction. There are thousands of medications available at the local discount store that will preserve the health of every organ in the body and do not require costly visits to a doctor. Indeed, these medications are so effective that their manufacturers are willing to offer the buyer double their money back if the medication does not work. With respect to fitness, hundreds of devices are offered through television infomercials that absolutely guarantee weight loss and a beautiful body and that require neither dietary restrictions nor sweat.

Because the population of the United States is, with respect to issues of health and wellness, functionally illiterate, the scams artists selling fradulent medical treatments and drugs continue to thrive and grow rich. Nobody buys full-page newspaper ads or 30 minute infomercials on television with the intention to lose money. They are growing rich off of people who do not understand how to critically evaluate their clames. Advertisements often have endorsements from persons with the initals "MD" after their names. What these ads do no reveal is that thos "doctors" are generally employees of the company whose product they are shilling. The purveyors of what can only be called "fraud" rely on the ignorance of the American public for their success.

The problems, such as they are, with "socialized medicine" arise not from the fact that it is a system operated

That Guy Nurse

by government but from the fact that, to some degree at least, it may still be driven with a primary goal of reducing costs rather than of building and maintaining the health and wellness of its population. Three characteristics separate the government-run medical programs in most of the world outside of the United States from the American medical system. **First**, there is a much higher emphasis on education and prevention. **Second**, there is in many countries a de facto rationing of medical care. **Third**, there is a higher sense of individual accountability for health.

This vision holds for us a medical system that is a true not-for-profit enterprise in which physicians have as their primary responsibility to teach people to become informed and capable managers of their own health and well-being. It will be a system that provides physicians the opportunity to teach and that rewards physicians for healthy outcomes. It will be a system in which every person has the opportunity to be healthy and has the knowledge required to guide life's activities in directions that promote health.

4. Primary care physicians will be compensated, in addition to the compensation provided by patients, on a scale that recognizes their contributions to prevention and the long-term health and wellness of their patients.

It is a common business practice to reward those employees

Part IV: A Vision for the Future of Medial Practice in the U.S.

whose skills and efforts contribute to the success of the business. It is not, however, common in medicine to single out and then reward those doctors whose skills and efforts contribute to the health and wellness of their patients. On the contrary, the doctors to receive the highest recognition and the greatest financial rewards tend to be those whose skills and efforts restore patients following illness or injury to whatever level of health may be possible. So just as businesses have found it profitable and appropriate to reward employees who excel in their contributions to the goals of the business, primary care physicians who demonstrate excellence in the task of working with patients to attain and maintain good health will be recognized and rewarded.

Shortly after I began my nursing career, I met a young doctor. He told me with some bitterness that during his years in medical school, he learned how to practice medicine, but when he came into the real world, he was simply not allowed to practice the medicine he had learned. The primary care physician is trained not just to diagnose sicknesses and injuries and then to develop a plan of care, often including referrals to specialists, but to be a person who, based upon knowledge of the patient, of the patient's values, and the patients' wishes, can provide information that can lead the patient to becoming knowledgeably proactive on behalf of the goal of personal health and wellness. Currently the primary care physician is simply not given the time required to listen to, to learn about, and to teach his patients. The one thing that those who pay for medical care will not pay for is the patient's time with the doctor. In fact, an accelerating trend in primary care medicine is to put patients in the care of nurse practitioners or physicians assistants, people with considerably less training and who cost considerably less than actual physicians.

While it is easy to place a value on a surgical procedure or on a medication, it is far more difficult to place a value on something that has been prevented. It's easy to cost out an open heart surgery but very difficult to measure the value of preventing the need for that surgery. However, as a growing number of businesses are discovering, as they endeavor to promote the health of their employees, it is possible to measure a return on investment by simply looking at the historical track record of illnesses and injuries and comparing that to the current record. It can certainly be argued that the past does not provide definitive guidance as to the present or future. But it is not unreasonable to assume that if, having instituted actions aimed at a specific preventative outcome—for example, the reduction of blood pressure or cholesterol levels—and then finding that these values have lowered, that these results are the product of those actions. And to the degree that one can objectively relate high blood

Part IV: A Vision for the Future of Medial Practice in the U.S.

pressure and elevated cholesterol to instances of heart attack and coronary disease, it is possible to place a value on these prevention activities.

This vision holds out a medical system that has become a true healthcare system by placing priority—and thereby incentives—on the building of health and wellness. It recognizes that the fundamental vehicle for achieving this outcome is the primary care physician and his relationship to his patients. It holds before us a medical system that identifies the dollar value of prevention, and then rewards those who, operating within the system, achieve a reduction in illness and injury and an increase in health and wellness.

5. Care for chronic medical conditions whose causes lie outside the control of patients (for example, Type 1 diabetes) will be provided by the single payer, again with the understanding that the patient will be financially responsible for that care to the extent determined by the patient's ability to pay.

There are many chronic medical conditions that, for many reasons, are not the fault of the persons who experience them. Down syndrome, Type 1 diabetes, a wide variety of birth defects, and the products of some accidents and environmental actions are examples of the kinds of things that can cause a person to have a long-term need for medical care. To the degree that the individual experiencing one or more of these conditions is, so to speak, innocent, needed medical care will be provided through the single-payer system. This is consistent with current practice to provide medical assistance to persons who are rendered disabled. In this vision, to be consistent with the principle of holding persons accountable for their health, only limited support, if any, will be available to those who brought their medical condition on themselves. Current medical practice requires that individuals and families who experience the kinds of chronic conditions described above must either bankrupt themselves before Medicaid has an obligation to provide support, or they must literally go into the community to beg for the funding needed.

The assessment of the degree of culpability of a patient—and thereby the extent to which support will be given for treatment—is going to be a very difficult and challenging matter. It will be argued that it is wrong to deny an individual treatment for sickness or injury, but that is exactly what happens today when people, however blameless for their condition, cannot receive needed care without facing bankruptcy or having to go into the community to beg for money.

Part IV: A Vision for the Future of Medial Practice in the U.S.

6. Employers will be released from any obligation to pay the costs of medical care for their employees or employee's families.

This will remove the temptation to take actions to reduce medical liability through termination of employees with chronic conditions or through hiring people on a part-time basis to avoid having to provide medical coverage.

The United States is alone in the world in having created a medical system whose primary source of funding is the employer. This system and this means of payment came into existence a little more than a half a century ago, a time when the costs of providing medical care were infinitesimally smaller than they are today. There were at that time very few medications, and surgeries were limited to procedures that today would almost entirely be done on an outpatient basis. The tools of diagnosis were the stethoscope and the blood pressure cuff. In those days, it was simply not possible to run up massive and ruinous bills for medical care. Thus it was relatively easy for America's businesses, under pressure from the unions, to agree to provide medical care as an employee benefit.

Today, though, the costs of the medical benefit to employers have become ruinous. At this time approximately $1500 of the cost of a car made by an American manufacturer

That Guy Nurse

is attributed to the costs of the medical benefit. This fact alone renders American automobile manufacturers unable to compete in the world market, and the result is that companies are shutting down plants and releasing tens of thousands of workers who, ironically, now have no medical benefits whatever.

For decades, employers, both private and governmental, offered increasing medical benefits in lieu of salary increases. Today they face an obligation to pay for medical care the cost of which far exceeds anything that they did or could have anticipated when they guaranteed the benefit.

This vision foresees a future in which the combination of requiring that individuals pay the costs of primary care, on a sliding fee scale based on ability to pay, and with the governmental single payer assuming costs that exceed the ability of individuals or families to pay for medical care, employers will be released from any obligation or expectation of participation. At the same time, and consistent with the current expectation that employers have an obligation to see to the safety of their employees while on the job (with the oversight of the Occupational Health and Safety Administration [OSHA]), employers may be expected to provide both programming and opportunities to inform and encourage employees about the maintenance of health and wellness.

Part IV: A Vision for the Future of Medial Practice in the U.S.

7. Decisions to forsake treatment aimed at cure and to initiate palliative care will be make by physician panels, with patients and families having the opportunity, should they disagree with a panel decision, to both appeal and/or to assume the costs of care.

You'll recall that in Chapter 12, I talked about the 72-year-old farmer who'd had a massive stroke after open-heart surgery and was comatose. His neurologist said that rehabilitation was not a reasonable possibility, and he recommended that all hydration be terminated and that the patient be allowed to die. Shortly afterward the patient's cardiologist met with the family and began rehydration because it's "what the family wanted." The farmer recovered and was discharged, still comatose, to a nursing home.

This scenario is repeated time after time in hospitals across the country. Although many physicians, perhaps a majority, are willing to counsel a course of palliative care— keeping the patient free of pain but withholding medications and treatments that would keep the patient alive—there continue to be many physicians who will not consider this option. Physicians and medical institutions that have a financial interest in providing ongoing care and a public that does not understand the limitations of medical care—and where the patient or family incurs no financial obligation for the continued treatment even though there is no reasonable expectation of recovery—lead to an increasingly frequent occurrence of futile care. This care is massively expensive in terms both of suffering and of dollars.

Conclusion

Remember, the above is a vision. Almost daily changes are taking place in Washington, in state capitals, in businesses, and in the institutions of American medicine. Some of these changes move us toward the realization of the vision. For example, the health care reform legislation passed in 2010 would eliminate the right of insurance companies to deny coverage on the basis of pre-existing conditions. Other parts of that legislation move us away from the vision, for example, the removal of the public option that would have given individuals the right to purchase insurance from the government. Thus, the for-profit private insurance sector remains in place and is even reinforced by the requirement that some 30 million people purchase insurance.

This vision is centered on two ideas. First, that each person is ultimately responsible for being well and healthy while acting as the chief executive officer of his or her life. Second, primary care medicine can and must be the heart of the American medical system. Any and all proposed changes in that system must be judged in terms of whether or not they enhance or damage the relationship between the

Part IV: A Vision for the Future of Medial Practice in the U.S.

primary care doctor and his patients.

notes:

_____

_____

_____

_____

_____

_____

_____

_____

_____

_____

_____

_____

That Guy Nurse

Epilog

Well, that's about it. The American medical system is broken.

Each and every day is it a part of our lives, sometimes for good and sometimes for bad. It is going to take a lot of time to fix it. It will probably take more time than most of the readers of this book have left to them. Yet it is the system we have and we're going to have to live with it.

> March 1965. Montgomery, Alabama. 25,000 marchers have concluded a walk from Selma, Alabama, to the state capitol in Montgomery on behalf of the rights of black people to vote. They are gathered in front of one of the capitol building. The flagpole on top of the capital displays a Confederate flag. The only American flag is on a small flagpole behind the capital in a parking lot.
>
> Martin Luther king addresses the assembled throng. His speech concludes with this: "I stand before you this afternoon with the conviction that segregation is on its deathbed in Alabama, and the only thing uncertain is how costly the segregationists and Wallace (the Governor of Alabama) will make the funeral.

Like the struggle for civil rights, which consumed so much time and so many lives, the struggle to rebuild the American medical system is one in which we, the patients, shall overcome. The only question is how much the medical corporations—the health systems, their hospitals and clinics, the insurance companies, the pharmaceutical companies and the companies that manufacture medical equipment—are going to make the funeral cost. It will be an expensive funeral but it is the funeral that can and must one day be held.

In the meantime we have to deal with the system as it is. It is a system that will keep us alive. It will not allow us to die. But when we come to understand that the foundations of health lie largely in the choices that we make, we gain immeasurably in the odds that after 90 to 95 years we will die but we will die having enjoyed health and well-being for all of that time. To a degree in far greater than any prior time in all of human history we have before us not only the opportunity but indeed the possibility of lifelong health.

It is my hope, indeed my prayer, that this book will help you, the reader, to understand how the system works and, in that understanding, to know how to make it work for you. Having spent 23 years working in a hospice and after 15 years as a registered nurse, I have seen too much unnecessary suffering and death. I have seen suffering and death that could have been averted if only patients had understood how they and their doctors can, working in a professional partnership, become powerful agents of health.

And so, I send this book forth hoping that it will make a difference, a good difference for you and for all who read it.

Thank you.

John Shier
thatguynurse

Appendix: Resources You Can Use

There is a vast literature available on the topics of health and wellness, of diet and exercise, of stress and relaxation, of stretching and balance. There are books and Web sites on yoga and meditation and Reiki and homeopathy and naturopathic medicine. So rather than providing a long list of books, articles, and Web sites, I want to encourage each reader to set off on his or her own exploration of these materials.

One of the first discoveries you'll make is that much of the available material is either wrong and/or fraudulent. It is a good test of one's medical literacy to be able to sort the wheat from the chaff. The simple but sad fact is that there is money to be made by promising the general public that a proffered product is almost miraculously effective in achieving weight loss, in preventing heart disease and cancer, or in effectively dealing with any of the health-related things that we fear, on the one hand, or hope to achieve, on the other.

The first and most important step in identifying the genuine from the false is to demand to "see the science." Before entrusting one's health and wellness to one or more of the myriad "scams" purporting to be medically sound, the Professional Patient will devote the time and energy necessary to understanding that any proposed "miracle" cure or treatment is well-based in the kind of scientific inquiry whose results are published in any of a number of reputable peer-reviewed journals.

Therefore, I want to suggest as excellent sources of information only a few resources that I have studied and found to provide accurate information and help. These resources can be gateways to the universe of good information. They are starting points. The rest is up to you.

Diet and Nutrition:

On the Web go to www.mypyramid.gov.

This site offers a great deal of information specifically tailored to the inquirer's gender, age, weight, and activity level. It contains the best scientifically validated information.

Eat, Drink, and Be Healthy by Walter C. Willett, MD

Dr. Willett's book may be the best book on nutrition available today. It is highly readable and contains, in addition to a wealth of information on diet, a section containing healthy recipes. Dr. Willett also offers a different food pyramid. It is instructive to compare the pyramid offered on "my pyramid.gov" with Dr. Willett's.

Your Medical Record:

No one should leave home (or even be home for that matter) without carrying a medical identification card. Nobody plans to have a medical emergency, but they happen. And when they happen, you will enter the medical system. Unless the system knows a great deal about you and you medical history, you have placed yourself at risk. Either procedures will be performed and medications given that, in the absence of your medical history, can be useless or, worse, damaging, or procedures and medications will be withheld when you should have received them. Either way, you are at risk.

My own experience tells me that I am utterly incapable of relating my medical history, my allergies, my blood type, and my medications and their schedule without prompting. Imagine how bad I (or anyone else) would be when sick or injured or in shock. Just try it yourself. Without notes or outside assistance, relate your complete medical history, your medications and schedule, etc. Then check your recollections against the record. You will be amazed.

Go to www.medids.com. Scroll down until you see an image of a wallet card on the left margin. Click on it. Follow the prompts to create your personal medical identification card. When it is printed, cut it out, fold it over, and have it laminated. It should be in your wallet or purse at all times next to your driver's license. Be sure to update it when your medical history changes, such as when a new medication is ordered or an old one discontinued. Worse than providing no information is providing wrong information.

Have spouse, children, parents, and anyone else you care about make their own cards, too.

Topic-based Information on Health, Wellness, and Medicine:

Harvard University and the Mayo Clinic both offer excellent Web sites containing a wealth of information, general and specific, on almost any health-related topic. Each site offers topic lists as well as an opportunity to request information on any specific topics in which you have interest.

www.health.harvard.edu

www.mayoclinic.com

Becoming medically literate will not be easy. It will require time and attention. Why make such an investment? It is your life and health that is on the line. As explained in the text of this book, living long is almost guaranteed by the American medical system. Living healthy all that time is up to you. To accomplish that end, you must learn about health and then put into practice the things you have learned. It will not be easy. Yet it is so sad to see how many people only become "experts" on heart disease, cancer, diabetes, depression, and other horrible conditions only when they or a loved one has become a victim.

It is true that knowledge is power. For us, the power is the power to prevent disease and disability as well as to promote high levels of health and wellness. Not too shabby, I say.